K·I·S·S

DK

The Only Guides You'll Ever Need!

THIS SERIES IS YOUR TRUSTED GUIDE through all of life's stages and situations. Want to learn how to surf the Internet or care for your new dog? Or maybe you'd like to become a wine connoisseur or an expert gardener? The solution is simple: just pick up a K.I.S.S. Guide and turn to the first page.

Expert authors will walk you through the subject from start to finish, using simple blocks of knowledge to build your skills one step at a time. Build upon these learning blocks and by the end of the book, you'll be an expert yourself! Or, if you are familiar with the topic but want to learn more, it's easy to dive in and pick up where you left off.

The K.I.S.S. Guides deliver what they promise: simple access to all the information you'll need on one subject. Other titles you might want to check out include: Playing Guitar, Weight Loss, Pregnancy, Gambling, Feng Shui, and many more to come.

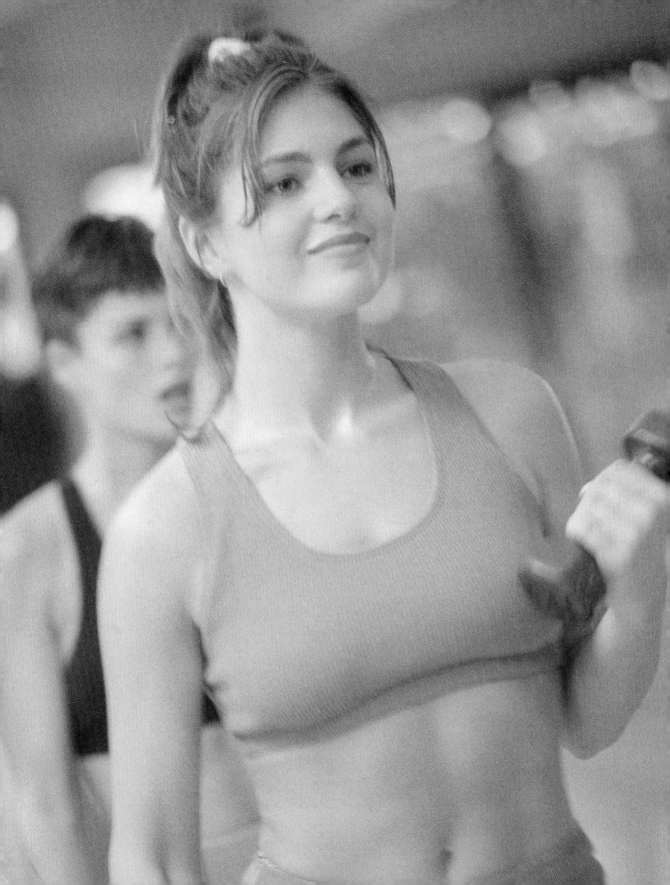

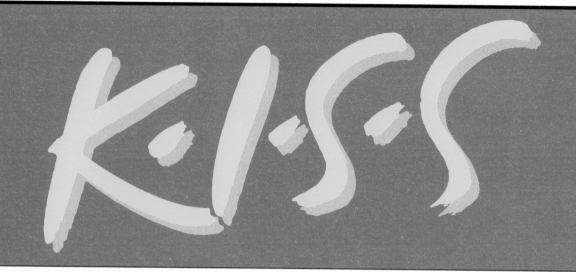

K·I·S·S

GUIDE TO

Fitness

MARGARET HUNDLEY PARKER

Foreword by **Rita Trieger**
Editor-in-Chief, *Fit Magazine*

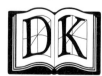

A Dorling Kindersley Book

LONDON, NEW YORK, MUNICH,
MELBOURNE, DELHI

Dorling Kindersley Limited
Project Editor Julian Gray
Art Editor Martin Dieguez

Managing Editor Maxine Lewis
Managing Art Editor Heather McCarry
Production Heather Hughes

Category Publisher Mary Thompson

Produced for Dorling Kindersley by **Cooling Brown**
9–11 High Street, Hampton, Middlesex TW12 2SA

Creative Director Arthur Brown
Senior Editor Amanda Lebentz

Art Editors Pauline Clarke, Elly King
Editor Patsy North

First published in Great Britain in 2002 by
Dorling Kindersley Limited
80 Strand, London
WC2 0RL

A Penguin Company

2 4 6 8 10 9 7 5 3 1

Copyright © 2002 Dorling Kindersley Limited.
Text copyright © 2002 Margaret Hundley Parker

A CIP catalogue record for this book is available from the British Library.

ISBN 0 7513 3528 2

Colour reproduction by ColourScan, Singapore
Printed and bound by MOHN media and Mohndruck GmbH, Germany

For our complete catalogue visit

www.dk.com

Contents at a Glance

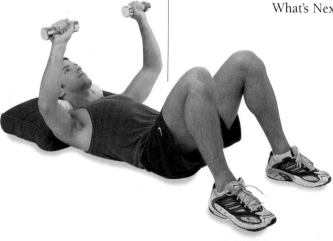

CONTENTS

PART ONE *Fitness Basics*

CHAPTER 1 Why Get Fit?   22

CHAPTER 2 Get Motivated   36

PART TWO Getting Fit

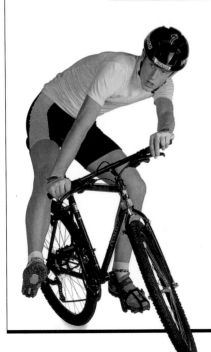

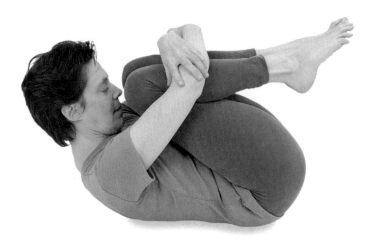

PART FOUR Fitness Essentials

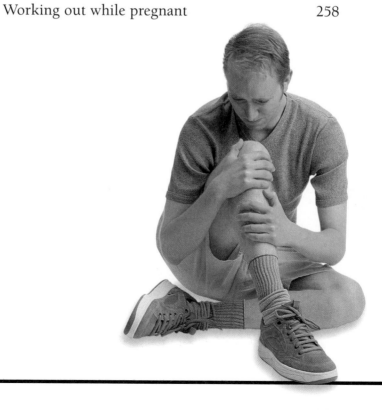

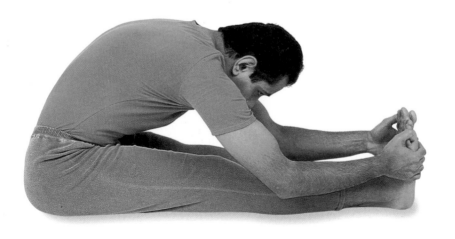

CHAPTER 20 *What's Next?*

Appendices

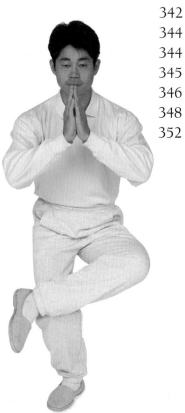

Foreword

WOULDN'T IT BE GREAT *if we could get into shape as quickly as we seem to get out of it? Or if there were a pill we could take that would miraculously melt away excess fat? Unfortunately, no one's ever been able to find a magic formula for keeping fit. Fitness must come from effort, discipline, and motivation.*

For a lot of people, the hardest part is finding the time to get fit. It's not easy to get your body moving after a hectic day at the office or an afternoon of running after toddlers. Maybe you're too exhausted to drive to the gym after work or there's no one around to look after the children; and even if you could find the spare hour here or there – you just don't know where to begin.

If this sounds all too familiar, know that you're not alone. I've been a personal trainer for many years and I've heard just about every excuse – legitimate or otherwise – a person can think of for not exercising. The one thing I know for certain is that once a person really wants to be fit and makes the decision to commit to a healthy lifestyle, they're in it for life. That's because exercise truly is a natural high. It gives you energy, self-esteem, helps you look and feel younger, helps you sleep better, relieves stress, and can ward off some diseases. Who wouldn't want to feel this good?

Some people may be too self-conscious to walk into a gym, while others may feel they just don't know enough fitness basics such as: What exactly is aerobics? What's a BMI? Why do I have to stretch? How much water should I drink? If this is what's been stopping you, then the K.I.S.S. Guide to Fitness is the perfect guide to a new, fit and healthy you.

I've had the pleasure of working with Margaret Parker for several years and her friendly personality shines through every chapter of this comprehensive fitness guide. Margaret addresses every aspect of exercise in simple, easy-to-understand terminology on every subject from how to get started and stay motivated, to the best ways to burn calories, choose a gym, eat healthily, and achieve a balanced diet.

You'll also find useful training suggestions, simple workouts, gym class descriptions, a future trends report, and tips on how to avoid basic injuries. This is one fitness book you shouldn't be without – you'll find yourself referring to it over and over again. I recommend it not only to beginners, but to seasoned gym-goers who are looking to take the next step on their fitness journey.

RITA TRIEGER
EDITOR-IN-CHIEF, *FIT MAGAZINE*

Introduction

WELCOME TO A FRESH APPROACH to fitness. If you've felt too overwhelmed or unmotivated to get in shape, then this is the book for you. The K.I.S.S. Guide to Fitness is different from other books on fitness because, basically, it's more fun. The focus of this book is to inform you about fitness and exercise and to give you the inside scoop from the fitness world.

The most important information about exercise and fitness is that it doesn't need to be a chore. It can be exciting. Let's face it, if it's not enjoyable, why do it? I'll give you all kinds of options so you can find a fitness routine that is perfect for you. As you probably already know, adding a little exercise to your routine can enrich your life in so many ways. We'll start off with simple methods to include movement in your daily life. Then we'll slowly move on to more challenging exercises. It's easy to get started when you break down your exercise programme into simple increments.

Staying fit is more important now than ever before. Many of our jobs don't require any physical exertion, so we have to make an effort to work exercise into our busy lives. And after all, these bodies of ours were made to move.

From my years of experience as a fitness writer and enthusiast, I'm well equipped to bring you all the news of latest trends as well as the old tried-and-true methods of getting in shape. I've always enjoyed exercise, but I know how it feels when work and life keeps us out of the gym for too long; so I'll share with you the tricks I've learned to stay motivated and keep it interesting.

Dive in. Together we'll stay fit and healthy.

Margaret Hundley Parker

MARGARET HUNDLEY PARKER

What's Inside?

THE INFORMATION in the K.I.S.S. Guide to Fitness *is arranged so that you learn the basic elements of a workout before moving on to toning specific areas of the body and developing an exercise programme to suit you and your lifestyle.*

PART ONE

In Part One, we'll take a look at the benefits of exercise and learn tips on how to get motivated. I'll also explain what to expect at the gym – from the machines to classes to gym etiquette. Learn about the different kinds of gyms and find the best one for you. We'll also go through some gear you'll need to get started. And, if there's no place like home, I'll help you set up your home gym.

PART TWO

In Part Two, we'll examine the basic elements of a workout – why it's important to warm up, stretch, work out, and cool down. We'll also get into some aerobic workouts and some lengthening and strengthening with exercises like yoga and Pilates. Then we'll muscle in on some tips for weight training.

PART THREE

In Part Three, it's time to get down to work and sweat. I'll give you a rundown of the muscles that you're going to be using and working on, and explain various ways to tone up the upper body, the lower body, and the midsection. We'll also go through a few simple all-over body exercise blasts.

PART FOUR

In Part Four we'll explore other aspects of fitness such as nutrition, treating injuries, exercise for travellers, and getting over an exercise hump. Also, we'll reassess our fitness goals and see how things are coming along. Finally, we'll take a sneak peak into the future of fitness.

The Extras

THROUGHOUT THE BOOK, *you will notice a number of boxes and symbols. They are there to emphasize certain points I want you to pay special attention to, because they are important in helping you get on the right fitness track. Here are the icons and what they mean:*

Very Important Point

This symbol means listen up. Here's some vital information that you'll need.

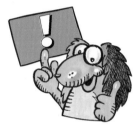

Complete No-No

Don't do it! This is a warning of something to avoid.

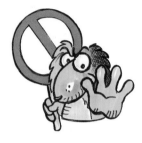

Getting Technical

When the information is about to get detailed or a little more complex, here's the heads-up to read carefully.

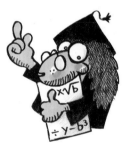

Inside Scoop

Here I'll let you in on anything from my experience in fitness that I think will help you understand.

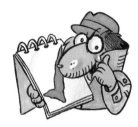

You'll also find some little boxes that include information I think is important, useful, or just plain fun.

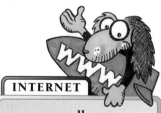

Trivia...

These are simply fun, quirky titbits about any aspect of fitness that I hope will add to your enjoyment and understanding.

DEFINITION

*Here I'll **define** any jargon or other health and fitness words that you need to know. You'll also find a Glossary at the back of the book with all the health and fitness lingo.*

INTERNET

www.dk.com

I think the Internet is a great resource, so I've pre-surfed for you and here I'll give you the lowdown on the fun fitness web sites I've discovered.

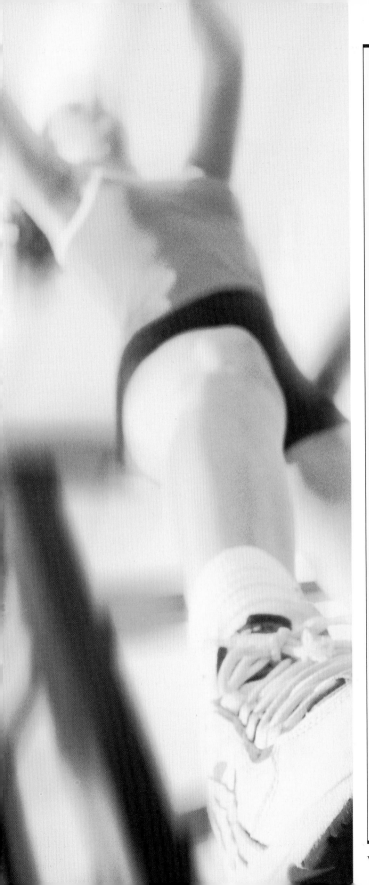

PART ONE

WHEN YOU'RE FIT, YOU HAVE MORE ENERGY FOR LIFE

FITNESS BASICS

IF YOU'RE NOT FEELING FIT, don't worry; you are not alone. Our society has made it very easy for us not to move too much. That's why we have to take matters into our own hands. *Getting in shape* can make you look and feel better and can help you *live a longer, healthier life*. If you're thinking, yes, but how? … read on.

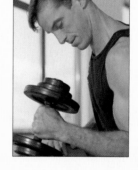

It's very simple to start a healthy lifestyle. First, we'll take a look at ways to add exercise into your daily life. Then, we'll assess your fitness situation and learn to *get motivated* – by setting goals, getting a partner, keeping a fitness diary, and, of course, rewarding yourself. We'll tell you what to expect at the gym, including a rundown of equipment and classes. Plus, we'll show you how to set up the home gym – whether you have a shoebox flat or a huge house. Best of all, we're going to help you have *fun* while getting *fit*!

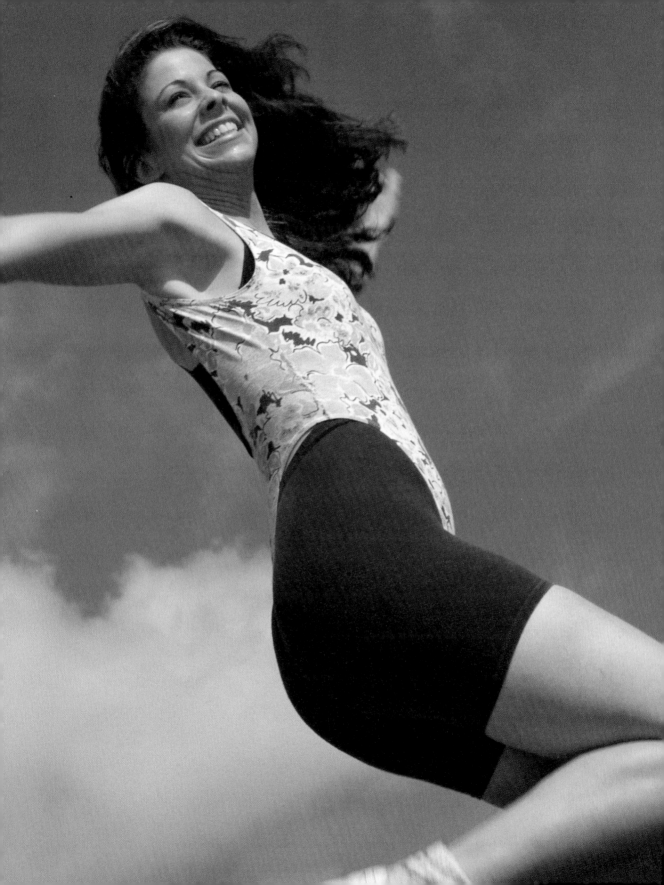

Chapter 1

Why Get Fit?

CONGRATULATIONS! Just by opening this book, you've made the decision to learn about fitness. It's the first step towards feeling great and enjoying a long, healthy life. Did you know that the hardest part is getting started? Learning about fitness is the right way to find the perfect regimen for your personal lifestyle. In this chapter, we'll take a look at the history of physical activity and learn why our bodies were created to move. We'll learn why it's extra important for us to find time to exercise these days and how exercise can help keep our weight under control, prevent disease, and keep our hearts happy.

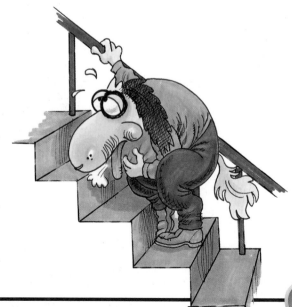

In this chapter...

✓ A brief history

✓ Physical benefits

✓ Psychological benefits

REGULAR EXERCISE HELPS KEEP YOU HEALTHY, TRIM, AND HAPPY

A brief history

STAYING IN GOOD PHYSICAL SHAPE *was not always the challenge that it is today. The human body was designed for a lot more physical activity than modern people need to survive. Nature and evolution have prepared us for a lifestyle very different from the one that most of us lead. The body that was made to live off the land, to roam from place to place, and to hunt is the same body that now has only to lift a finger to order dinner with a mouse click.*

While we don't have much information on the health of humans from the very early days, observations of the few remaining nomadic groups who live much as did our ancestors reveal that they have a higher level of physical activity and are leaner and more free of chronic diseases than are people in developed countries. If it's so natural and healthy, why did we stop being active?

Living off the land

The nature of our civilization has been changing slowly from active to more sedentary. During the Agricultural Age – a mere 10,000 years ago – people began to settle down, grow crops, and keep domesticated animals. Although these people were no longer nomadic, the demands on their energy were very high. Just ask anyone who lives on a farm!

In the mid-18th century, as advances such as the steam engine and factory machinery led society into the Industrial Revolution, more people moved from farms to the cities; but daily life was still very physically demanding. There weren't as many options for transportation, so most people walked to work. And in the cities more people had to walk up more stairs.

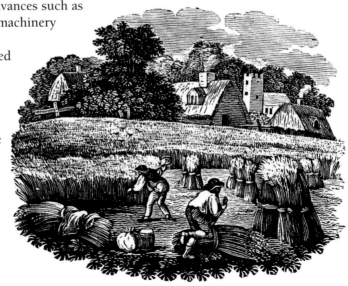

■ **Harvesting crops** *without machinery was physically very demanding, so people who worked the land tended to be strong and fit.*

The big slowdown

When did we become a sedentary society? Since the Technological Age, which started after World War II and still continues, there has been a rapid growth in labour-saving devices for home and employment and even for work in the garden. Just think about the changes that have occurred in your lifetime.

Many activities that required sweat and muscle now require only a finger to dial the phone or click the mouse. Now you don't even have to leave your room to buy anything from dinner to a pair of shoes to a new car. Dirty dishes? Put them in the dishwasher. Need to rake the leaves? Get a leaf-blower. Need to give a colleague a memo? Don't get up from your chair; e-mail it across the room. Instead of going to the local cinema, just put your favourite DVD on the home entertainment system. All these modern conveniences of our highly technological society discourage physical activity in many ways, and it's easier than ever before to remain sedentary.

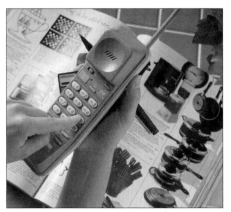

■ **Being able to buy goods** *from the comfort of your own home has reduced the need to go out shopping.*

While participation in regular physical activity in developed countries gradually increased during the '60s, '70s, and early '80s, it levelled off in the '90s. In fact, current studies find that today almost 50 per cent of British adults are overweight and out of shape.

Because of all these wonderful labour-saving devices, we now have to make a special effort to exercise. Although the benefits of exercise have been well publicized, most people still don't do it. So if you're not working out regularly, you are certainly not alone. Let's start the fitness revolution of the 2000s!

■ **Now that messages** *can be delivered via computer, there's no reason to get up and walk around at work. This makes exercising outside the office even more important.*

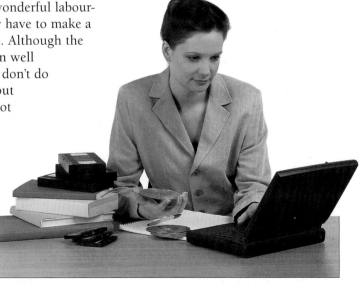

Physical benefits

WHY PUT ON THE TRACKSUIT *and go outside and run when it's so nice and cosy on the sofa? In a nutshell – why exercise? There are many well-known physical benefits, such as being able to do up the top button on your favourite pair of jeans without having to suck in your stomach. Most people begin an exercise programme in order to lose weight. Regular exercise does keep your weight down. This not only makes you look and feel better but is important for your health.*

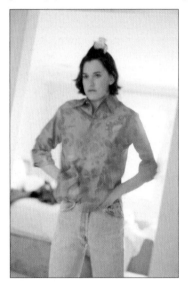

■ **Exercising will help you**
ease into, rather than squeeze into, those favourite jeans.

Being overweight not only makes those jeans uncomfortable, it also puts you at a greater risk of sickness and many diseases. People who are overweight have a greater chance of developing heart disease, diabetes, high blood pressure, stroke, arthritis, and fatigue. The best way to lose weight is by doing physical activity that makes you breathe hard, causing your body to burn **calories** faster.

DEFINITION

A **calorie** *is a unit of energy-producing potential equal to the amount of heat that is contained in food, and released when combined with oxygen from the body. In other words, burning calories means converting food into energy. When you burn calories, the food is used up and isn't stored as fat in the body.*

Muscle burns more calories than fat

The good news is that once you start exercising, it becomes easier to lose weight. By building muscle, you're ahead of the game because muscle burns more calories than fat, even when you're not exercising. After the workout, at rest, muscles still require more calories. That means that an active person with more muscle mass burns more calories just sitting there than does a sedentary person with less muscle. Please note that muscle weighs more than fat, so don't get discouraged if you're working out and not shedding a lot of weight. Instead of worshipping the mighty scales, pay attention to how your clothes fit.

Avoid unrealistic fad or crash diets. You may lose weight at first, but you're likely to gain it right back once you go off the diet.

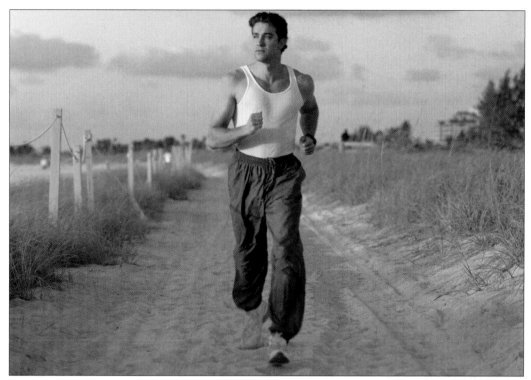

■ **Regular physical activity** *such as jogging is enormously beneficial as it helps maintain a healthy heart and circulation. Try to make some form of exercise part of your daily routine.*

You probably will lose weight if you eat only carrot sticks or take diet pills, but the best way to lose weight is by combining a good diet with exercise. Not only will you feel better, you'll see results faster. Diet without exercise tends to rob the body of lean muscle tissue and water, two vital parts of a healthy body. Choose a diet and exercise plan you can stick to long-term.

Besides keeping your weight under control, being physically active can save your life by making your heart healthy and happy. The leading causes of death in 1900 were diseases that are now controllable with modern medicine, such as pneumonia and tuberculosis.

In 1990, among the most common causes of death were heart disease and stroke, which are preventable through lifestyle choices – including being fit.

One of the most common causes of death in adults in developed countries is cardiovascular disease.

27

Why do aerobic exercise?

The term "aerobic exercise" refers to exercise that strengthens the heart. More specifically, aerobic exercise is activity that is sustained, repetitive, or rhythmic, that uses big muscle groups and is fairly light to heavy in intensity.

Aerobic exercise reduces high blood pressure and improves cardiovascular health. Imagine your arteries and veins as roads. Doing aerobic exercise is like paving the road so your blood can get around more easily. As your heart becomes stronger, it doesn't have to work as hard to pump blood through your body, thereby lowering your blood pressure. Physical exercise reduces the risk of heart disease by improving blood circulation throughout the body.

Another benefit of regular exercise is a stronger immune system – the system in your body that fights off sickness and disease. Even low to moderate exercise such as walking can make you more resistant to colds, flu, or other diseases because as you strengthen your body, you enhance your immune system's ability to fight infection.

Are you so busy that you don't have enough energy at the end of the day to hit the gym? That's not a good excuse. Exercise is invigorating. It's the gift that keeps on giving; the more you exercise, the more energy you have for everyday life.

INTERNET

www.justmove.org

To find out more about exercise and cardiovascular health, or to get daily news updates on health and fitness trends and breakthroughs, check out this web site by the American Heart Association.

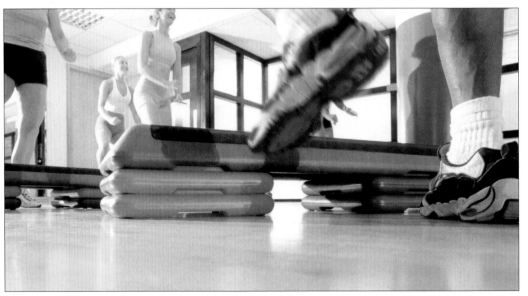

■ **Aerobic exercise** *works and strengthens the heart, helping your entire circulatory system function more efficiently, and reducing the risk of high blood pressure.*

Psychological benefits

EXERCISE FOR HAPPINESS! *Beyond having a swimsuit-ready body, developing grapefruit-sized muscles, or even having a happy heart, being* physically active improves your psychological health. Regular exercise improves your mood and makes you less likely to get depressed. It can also help you handle stressful situations calmly.

Relieve depression

Whether or not you're feeling blue, exercise can lift your mood and help you feel positive, even in times of adversity. Exercise alleviates depression by providing a natural antidepressant, boosting self-esteem, and enabling you to put things in perspective. Aerobic exercise forces oxygenated blood to the brain as well as to other parts of the body.

Have you ever heard of "runner's high"? It refers to the euphoric feeling that comes from the rush of endorphins that are released during vigorous exercise.

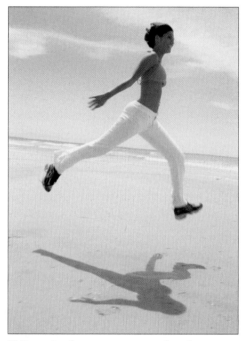

■ **Exercise boosts your mood** *and can actually make you feel like jumping for joy.*

When aerobic exercise gets blood flowing to the brain, this new blood changes the chemical makeup within the brain and can have the same effect as drugs prescribed for depression. Also, exercise triggers the release of endorphins, which are hormones that produce a sense of wellbeing and reduce stress.

When you're depressed, staring at the four walls of your room might seem like the answer. Alas, it is not. Getting out and moving around is the best thing you can do for yourself. It can change your outlook for the better. Even if all you feel like doing is walking – walk! Even minimal exercise can get you out of a rut, change your perspective, broaden your vision, even boost your self-esteem. Hey, you might get inspired to do more. Some psychologists and psychiatrists prescribe exercise to their patients and see good results. These patients often show improved mood and functioning.

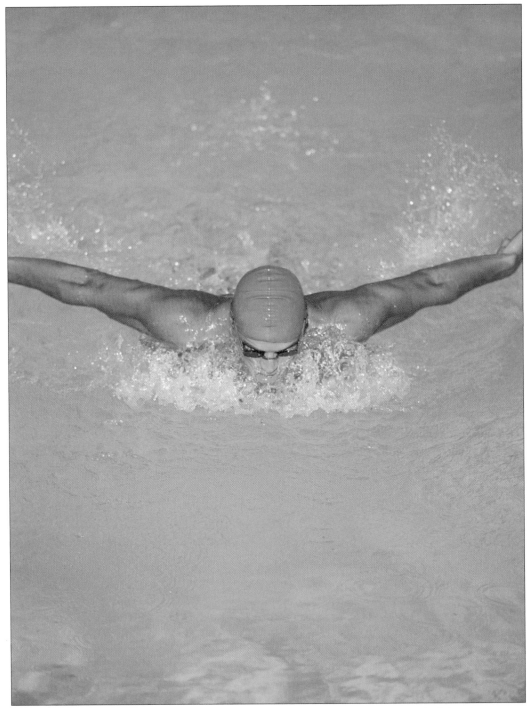

■ **Swimming is a great physical activity** *for people of all ages. Many swimmers find that focusing on their strokes as they do laps of the pool helps them relax mentally, too.*

A recent study conducted in America showed that exercise was more effective than drugs at relieving depression. The survey of 156 middle-aged patients found that those who exercised showed a significant improvement compared to those taking drugs, or a combination of drugs and exercise.

Squash stress with sit-ups

You're on a deadline and your computer has crashed. On the way home from work, you get a flat tyre. Instead of kicking your bumper or snapping at a loved one, jump on a bicycle. Lift weights. You'll feel better, and here's why:

Exercise is a great physical outlet for emotional stress. What happens to your body when you're stressed? How can exercise help? For one thing, stressful situations trigger your ancient "fight or flight" response. This can make your heart beat faster to make more blood and oxygen available. Aerobic activity keeps your heart in top shape and more able to handle the extra workload. Also, stress causes digestion to slow down to save energy. Physical activity enhances the digestive function, giving your gut a jump-start.

Whenever I feel overwhelmed with work or get stressed, I take a few minutes to run around the block. With a bit more time, I go to the gym. I inevitably come back refreshed and more able to focus. It's like magic!

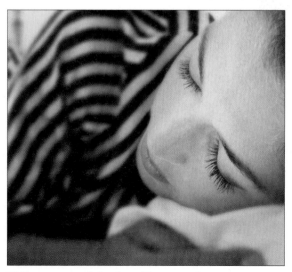

Sleep soundly

Have you ever flopped down on the bed at night only to stare wide-eyed into the darkness, haunted with thoughts from the day? Well, stress can cause insomnia. Have no fear – exercise can also help you sleep. If you have trouble sleeping, work out at least two or three hours before you go to bed. (You don't want to do a lot of strenuous exercise too close to bedtime.) Working out relieves muscle tension and wears you out physically, so it's easier to fall asleep. If it's the workday that stresses you out, try exercising in the morning before work.

■ **Rest assured** *that by taking some time out to exercise during the day, you'll sleep easy at night.*

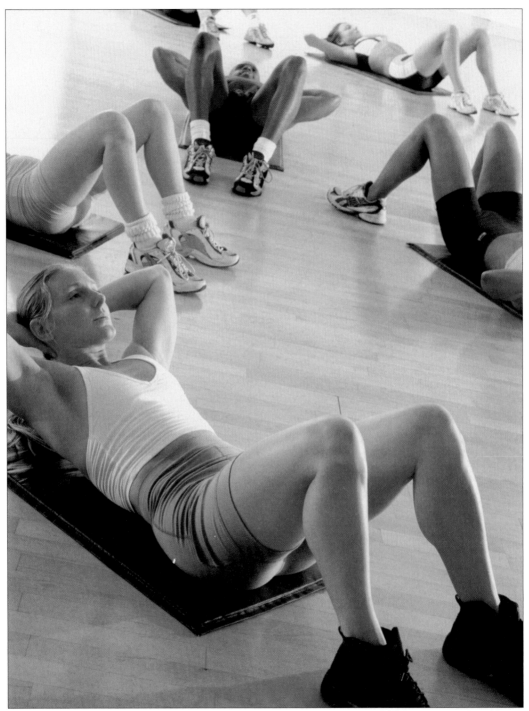

■ **It doesn't take long to feel the effects** *of exercise – in fact, it's possible to see a visible difference within a matter of weeks. So the sooner you start, the faster you'll feel better about yourself.*

Moves that make a difference

Here are my top ten ways to add movement to your daily routine:

1. **Take the stairs**: skip the lift or escalator and take the stairs once a day. If you have stairs at the office or at home, make it fun: put a sign-up sheet at the bottom of the stairs for everyone to sign when choosing to take the stairs

2. **Skip the parking space**: instead of circling the car park looking for that perfect space, park at the far end and walk. A few extra steps add up

3. **Walk or cycle instead of drive**: instead of putting the key in the ignition, put on your walking shoes or hop on your bicycle

4. **Go to the shops**: now that shopping can be a matter of clicking a mouse or dialling a phone, make an effort and go to the shops. Browse in a bookshop or walk a few extra laps around the shopping centre

5. **Clean the house**: yes, housework counts! Do your own housework instead of hiring someone (or not doing it at all). Wash the dishes by hand, sweep and mop the floor, or put clothes away

6. **Garden**: work in the garden, mow the grass (no, riding mowers don't count), prune, dig, pick up rubbish

7. **Watch television**: I can't lie; you're not going to get in shape by watching television. But if you must, sit up instead of lying down. Or better still, pedal on a stationary bike, stretch, or at least throw away the remote

8. **Stretch**: if you've been sitting for a long time, roll your shoulders backwards and forwards, roll your neck, stretch your arms out in front of you, and take a deep breath

9. **Fidget**: when talking on the phone, stand up and walk around. When sitting, twirl a pencil or pen, chew gum, or move your legs around

10. **Get out of your chair at the office**: walk down the hall instead of calling or e-mailing a colleague. Walk around the block at lunchtime. Try having a walking meeting with colleagues

Lift your mood

Although maximum benefits come with regular exercise and fitness, just one session can generate a relaxation response. You feel better even after a mellow workout, but the best way to get the mood-lifting effect is to do 20 minutes of aerobic exercise. (Remember, that means getting that heart beating.)

It is important, and sometimes difficult, to get some time on your own during the day. Exercise is a good way to get time to yourself, to think and put things in perspective. The process of repetitive motion, such as the one you perform with weightlifting or sit-ups, can provide a mind-clearing meditation.

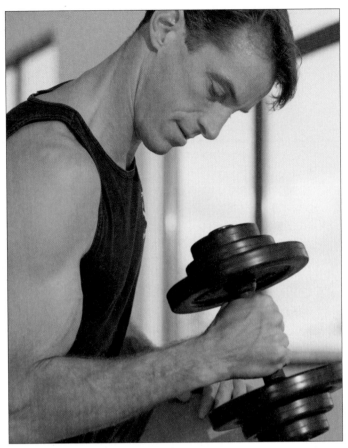

■ **Concentrating on maintaining** *repetitive movements such as lifting weights takes your mind off day-to-day problems.*

Of course, exercise also makes you feel better about yourself. It slims you down and tones you up, thereby boosting your self-confidence. Your body image plays a huge role in your overall mental health.

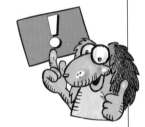

Simple ways to add more exercise to your daily routine

All this exercise sounds great – but who has time? Committing to an exercise programme can seem a bit overwhelming. Recent studies prove that even moderate movement, when done for as little as 30 minutes a day, can improve your health and reduce your chances of heart and other diseases.

The good news is that you don't even have to do it all at once. You can get your 30 minutes in with three 10-minute sessions or any other small increments you have time for. By making just a few changes in your daily routine, you can get that body moving and be well on your way to being fit.

Remember, just keep it simple. You don't have to sign up to run a marathon next week in order to start getting fit. Small changes in your daily routine can really add up.

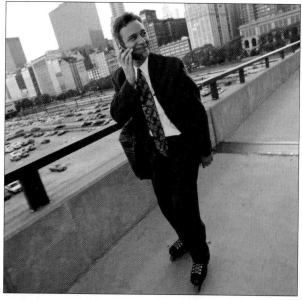

■ **Hectic schedules** *need not mean forgoing exercise – even if you can only manage 10 minutes on the skates between appointments, you'll feel the benefits.*

A simple summary

✔ Our bodies are designed to be physically active. Now that technological advances have made it very easy to lead a sedentary lifestyle, we have to make a special effort to exercise.

✔ Regular exercise can not only keep you slim and trim, it can get your heart healthy and prevent cardiovascular disease.

✔ Physical activity can alleviate depression and stress, help you sleep, and boost self-esteem.

✔ There are plenty of simple ways to add a little movement to your daily routine without having to change your entire lifestyle.

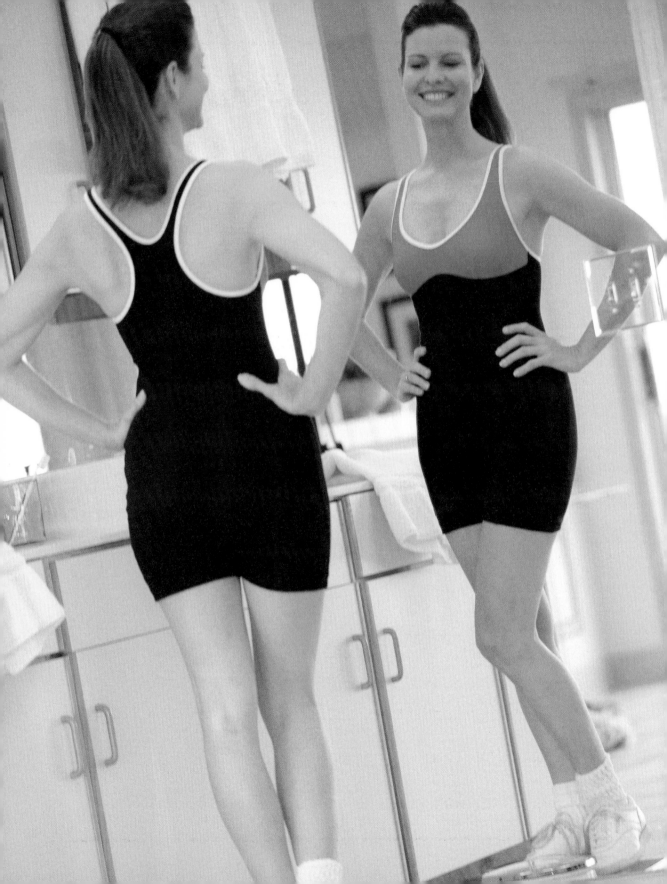

Chapter 2

Get Motivated

KNOW THYSELF. A vital aspect of any fitness programme is knowing your own capabilities and limitations. Evaluating your current weight and fitness level will not only help you get motivated, it will also help you figure out the best way to get in better shape. Your initial evaluation will establish your baseline so that once you start working out you can see your progress. In this chapter, you'll take a quiz to find out more about your body.

In this chapter...

✓ Assess your weight and fitness level

✓ Set realistic goals

✓ Be accountable

✓ Keep a fitness diary

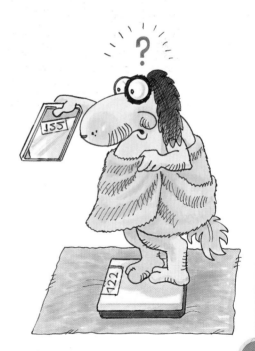

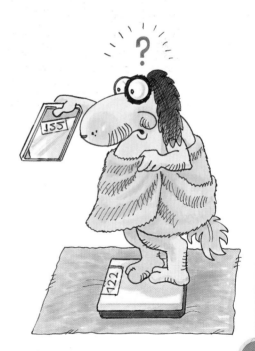

ASSESSING THE SHAPE YOU'RE IN NOW WILL START YOU ON THE ROAD TO FITNESS

Assess your weight and fitness level

EVALUATING YOUR CURRENT LEVEL *of fitness is the first step in finding an exercise programme that's right for you. If you're a seasoned runner, joining the local rambling club is unlikely to challenge you. If you haven't exercised in 10 years, deciding to train for a triathlon in 2 months will surely result in injury. Once you're aware of your capabilities and limits, you're more likely to find something you'll stick to, and you're less likely to be hurt.*

Besides helping to find an exercise programme you like, another reason to evaluate yourself and establish a baseline is so you can record your progress. On the following pages, we'll measure weight and body composition, waist-to-hip ratio, muscle strength, and flexibility. These are key elements to any fitness programme.

Weight assessment

Let's get the worst part over first. Weigh yourself and write it down. Before you get discouraged and run off with a box of chocolates, keep in mind that the number on the scales is not the ultimate measure of fitness. Many factors – genes that determine your body size and shape, age, gender, what you eat, and how much you exercise – affect your weight. Besides, muscle weighs more than fat.

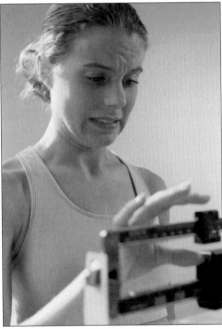

■ **Bite the bullet** *and find out how much you weigh. It may not be as bad as you think.*

INTERNET

www.fitlinxx.com

If you don't feel like doing the sums, log on to this fitness web site and go to the "Assess yourself – workout tools" section. Enter your height and weight, and the site will calculate your BMI for you.

To determine if you're at a healthy weight, it's important to figure out what your body composition is. In other words, how much of your weight is made up of fat and how much is dense (like muscles, bones, and organs)? The Body Mass Index, which measures your height and weight to calculate how much body fat you have, is an easy way to determine this.

CALCULATING YOUR BODY MASS INDEX

Find your BMI on this chart by looking for your height and weight and locating the box where the two columns meet. To calculate your BMI manually, simply divide your weight in kilograms by your height in metres squared. If you use the imperial system, multiply your weight in pounds by 704, then divide by the square of your height in inches. For example, if you weigh 162 pounds and are 69 inches (5 ft 9 ins) tall, your BMI is (162 x 704) ÷ (69 x 69) = 23.9. Refer to the key below to see how you shape up.

Height (in)

Weight (lb)	58	60	62	64	66	68	70	72	74	76	78	Weight (kg)
340	71	66	62	58	55	52	49	46	44	41	39	154
320	67	62	59	55	52	49	46	43	41	39	37	145
300	63	59	55	51	48	46	43	41	39	37	35	136
280	59	55	51	48	45	43	40	38	36	34	32	127
260	54	51	48	45	42	40	37	35	33	32	30	118
240	50	47	44	41	39	36	34	33	31	29	28	109
220	46	43	40	38	36	33	32	30	28	27	25	100
200	42	39	37	34	32	30	29	27	26	24	23	90
180	38	35	33	31	29	27	26	24	23	22	21	82
160	33	31	29	27	26	24	23	22	21	19	18	73
140	29	27	26	24	23	21	20	19	18	17	16	63
120	25	23	22	21	19	18	17	16	15	15	14	54
100	21	20	18	17	16	15	14	14	13	12	12	45
80	17	16	15	14	13	12	11	11	10	10	9	36
	147	152	157	163	168	173	178	183	188	193	198	

Height (cm)

KEY

COLOUR	BMI	
	Less than 18	Underweight
	18 – 24	Desirable weight
	25 – 29	Overweight
	30 – 40	Obese
	More than 40	Severely obese

That said, be aware that some people should not use the BMI (Body Mass Index) as an indicator of body composition. It's not a good measure for conditioned athletes, women who are pregnant or breastfeeding, preadolescent children, or sedentary elderly people.

There are other methods to determine your BMI, but these must be done professionally. One way is the "pinch test" in which the tester uses skin-fold callipers to pinch the skin and fat on various places of your body such as your thighs, back of your arms, and waist. The numbers on the callipers translate into your BMI.

Another way to determine BMI is the "tank test" in which you sit on underwater scales in a large tank, then submerge for 5 seconds. Your underwater weight is then translated into your BMI.

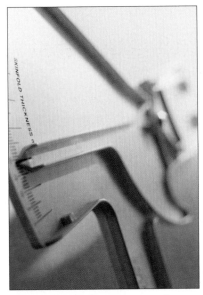

■ **Skin-fold callipers** *are used to measure the thickness of the fat layer under the skin.*

Waist assessment

TAPE MEASURE

Now it's time to get out the trusty measuring tape. You can do this yourself; no one else needs to know your measurements. We're just establishing a baseline here. It's no secret where on the body fat likes to accumulate – waist, thighs, buttocks, upper arms. Therefore, another way to assess your current state of physical fitness is by measuring your waist-to-hip ratio.

Where you store your fat is an important health factor. People who are heavier in the middle are more at risk for health problems such as hypertension, Type II diabetes, and heart disease – even when compared to people who are equally fat but whose fat is more evenly distributed.

Testing your muscle strength

Now it's time to put on some comfortable clothes and evaluate your muscle strength. An easy way to measure this at home is by measuring upper body and abdominal strength with push-ups and crunches. If you're evaluated professionally, you'll probably be asked to lift a variety of weights.

MEASURING YOUR WAIST-TO-HIP RATIO

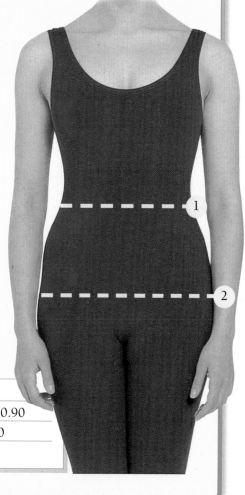

1 **Record your waist measurement**

While standing, exhale normally (but don't suck in your stomach). Measure your waist at the belly button and write down the number.

2 **Find the widest part of your hips**

Measure your hips at the widest point, going around the biggest part of your ... um, glutes.

3 **Now simply divide the two**

Divide the waist measurement by the hip measurement and voila! You've got your waist-to-hip ratio. For example, if your waist measures 87.5 cm (35 in) and your hips are 102.5 cm (41 in), divide 87.5 by 102.5 (35 by 41) and you get a waist-to-hip ratio of 0.85.

	WOMEN	MEN
Healthy:	Less than 0.80	Less than 0.90
Borderline:	0.80 to 0.85	0.90 to 1.0
Unhealthy:	Above 0.85	Above 1.0

If you haven't been exercising regularly, don't over-exert yourself. Do the best you can without causing any pain.

To measure upper body endurance, stretch out on the floor, belly down, and get in push-up position – hands below your shoulders and toes on the floor. (Women, who have less upper body strength than men, often choose the modified version with knees on the floor.)

Try to push yourself up, keeping a straight line from your neck to your knees or feet. Don't arch your back. Record how many you can do without resting or compromising form, and compare your performance to the chart below to see how you measure up.

The best way to test abdominal strength is to see how many sit-ups or crunches you can do. Here we'll measure crunches, which aren't quite as challenging as full-force sit-ups.

ASSESSING YOUR SCORE FOR PUSH-UPS

FEMALE FITNESS LEVEL

Age	Poor	Fair	Average	Good	Excellent
29 or younger	0–5	6–16	17–33	34–50	More than 50
30 to 39	0–3	4–11	12–24	25–40	More than 40
40 to 49	0–2	3–7	8–19	20–35	More than 35
50 to 59	0–1	2–5	6–14	15–30	More than 30
60 or older	0	1–2	3–4	5–20	More than 20

MALE FITNESS LEVEL

Age	Poor	Fair	Average	Good	Excellent
29 or younger	0–19	20–34	35–44	45–55	More than 55
30 to 39	0–14	15–24	25–34	35–45	More than 45
40 to 49	0–11	12–19	20–29	30–40	More than 40
50 to 59	0–7	8–14	15–24	25–35	More than 35
60 or older	0–5	5–9	10–19	20–30	More than 30

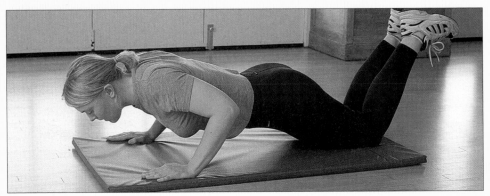

■ **Push-ups are a** *great way to measure your upper body strength. Women may choose to use the modified version with knees on the floor. Make sure you warm up first before starting the test.*

Skip the crunches if you have a bad back.

Lie on your back with your hands by your head. Bend your knees and keep your feet on the floor. Now, lift your upper body up so that your head, chest, and shoulder blades are off the floor, but your lower back remains touching the floor at all times. Return upper body to the floor; that's one crunch. Do as many as you can without pausing, and check yourself against the chart below.

ASSESSING YOUR SCORE FOR CRUNCHES

FEMALE FITNESS LEVEL

Age	Poor	Fair	Average	Good	Excellent
29 or younger	0–15	16–30	31–40	41–60	More than 60
30 to 39	0–10	11–15	16–35	36–50	More than 50
40 to 49	0–5	6–10	11–25	26–40	More than 40
50 to 59	0–2	3–5	6–20	21–30	More than 30
60 or older	0	1–3	4–9	10–20	More than 20

MALE FITNESS LEVEL

Age	Poor	Fair	Average	Good	Excellent
29 or younger	0–20	21–35	36–45	46–70	More than 70
30 to 39	0–15	16–20	21–40	41–60	More than 60
40 to 49	0–10	11–15	16–35	36–50	More than 50
50 to 59	0–5	6–10	11–25	26–40	More than 40
60 or older	0	1–5	6–15	16–30	More than 30

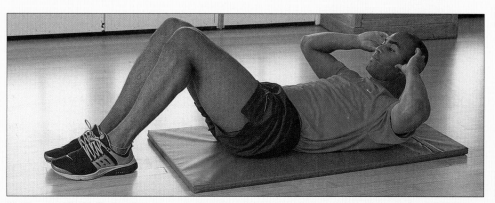

■ **The number of crunches** *you can do will give you a good idea of your abdominal strength. Keep your lower back touching the floor and do not pull at your neck at any time during the exercise.*

Testing your flexibility

Flexibility is an important, and often overlooked, aspect of being fit. Being flexible is more than just being able to bend over and touch your toes. Flexibility helps prevent injuries and enhances balance and co-ordination. Below are two quick flexibility tests. Before you begin them, warm up with a short walk or jog in place. Once you feel loose, you can begin.

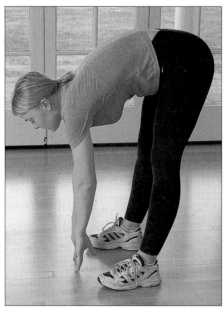

STEP 2

1 Stand up straight with your feet shoulder-width apart

2 Bend at the waist, reaching towards the floor without bending your knees

3 Note how far you can reach and write it down. (You may want to try this a few times and record your longest reach)

Verdict: If you can easily touch the floor, you have good flexibility here. If you can touch your toes, you're moderately flexible. If you can't reach the floor, you need to work on this.

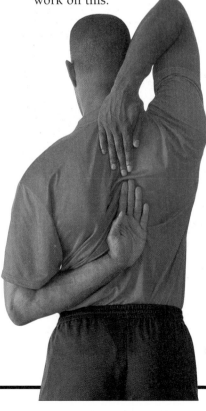

Next, test how flexible your shoulders are:

1 Take your right arm and reach down your back as far as you can

2 Reach your left hand up your back and try to touch your right hand

3 Try switching arms, reaching down with your left and up with your right

Verdict: If you can clasp your hands together easily, you have good flexibility in your shoulders. If you can bring your fingers close but without touching, you are moderately flexible. If your hands don't even come close, you're stiff in this area and might experience discomfort. Another useful measure of fitness is heart rate. We'll discuss heart rate in depth in Chapter 7.

STEP 2

Set realistic goals

NOW THAT YOU KNOW WHERE YOU ARE in the fitness game, *where do you want to be? Setting goals is an excellent way to keep yourself on track. If you set long- and short-term goals, you're more likely to stick to your exercise programme. Be sensible in setting up your exercise programme. Don't say, "I'm going to run two miles every day" if you hate running. Choose something you enjoy doing. And be very specific in setting goals. Ask yourself what exactly it is you want to happen (weight loss? firmer thighs?), when you want it to happen, and how you will know when it has happened. Make your goals realistic. If you reach for the impossible, you're bound to fail.*

Here are some examples of short-term goals:

● I will find an exercise partner
● I will check out the local gym
● I will walk for half an hour, three
 times this week
● I will quit smoking

Here are some examples of long-term goals:

● I will increase my cardiovascular
 strength
● I will lose 10 kg (22 pounds) (break
 this down into smaller goals)
● I will run 5 kilometres (3.1 miles)
● I will do 25 push-ups

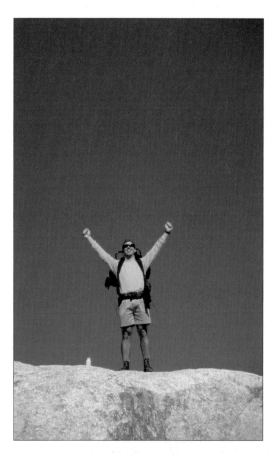

In general, a total exercise programme should include aerobic exercise, strengthening, and stretching. On the following pages, you'll find some guidelines to help you set appropriate goals.

■ **Setting goals** *helps you focus on what you want to achieve. Visualize yourself reaching a major milestone and imagine the satisfaction it will bring.*

How often?

To see any results, you should exercise two or three times a week at the very least. Don't go more than 2 days without exercising, if you can help it. If you're trying to lose fat, you should exercise at least 3 days a week for 20 minutes at a time. You can exercise more, but only if you're careful not to overtrain.

How much?

The optimal intensity required to produce benefits has been the subject of much study. It's nice to know that the fitness world has thankfully moved away from the "no pain, no gain" rhetoric of the '80s.

Exercise doesn't have to hurt to be effective.

You need to exert yourself only to 45-50 per cent of your maximum capability. This is a comfortable level at which most people improve physiological functioning – the functions of the body and all its parts – and overall health. Determine your own maximum capability by taking a *talk test*.

> **DEFINITION**
>
> *A **talk test** is a way to assess if you're working out too hard. If you can't easily carry on a conversation while exercising, then you should slow down. It's especially unsafe for beginners to continue above the conversation level.*

How long?

The relationship between duration and intensity is this: if you exercise at a very high intensity, such as running, the workout doesn't need to be as long. On the other hand, if you're working out at a lower intensity, such as walking, the duration should increase in order to get the benefits. In general, you get the maximum benefits if you exercise for at least 15 to 20 minutes. Unless you're in serious training mode, going hard for longer than an hour is not advised.

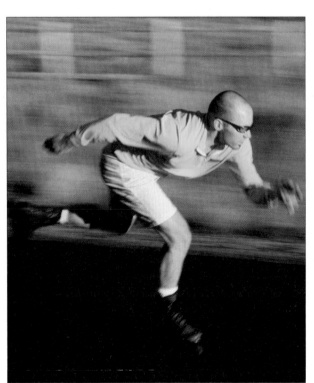

■ **A 20-minute session** *of reasonably vigorous exercise, such as in-line skating, is enough to bring about benefits.*

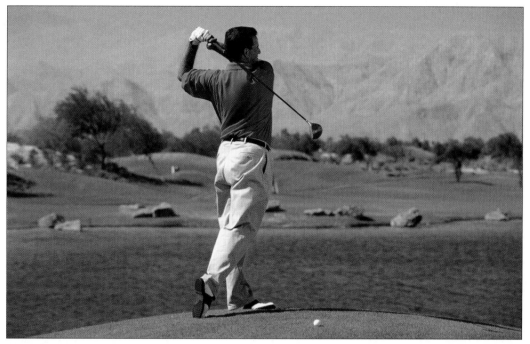

■ **A leisurely morning on the golf course** *can do as much to raise fitness levels as an intense 20-minute aerobic workout – provided you play a round on a regular basis.*

Which type?

The most important thing is that you find something you like, so you'll do it. If it's a 2-hour stroll through the park you love, then do that. Or if you'd rather go full steam ahead and spend the minimum time in an aerobics class or on the track, then go for it. A leisurely 4-hour golf game or a brisk 1-hour walk can provide the same effects for maintaining physical fitness. Please be assured that there is no best exercise. The one that's the best is the one you do regularly.

How to progress

When you start working out, begin at a level that's just above your daily routine and gradually increase the frequency, duration, and intensity. Although there are no hard-and-fast rules about how quickly to progress, it ordinarily takes 4 to 8 weeks to elevate your fitness level from low to high. In general, don't progress to a higher level more often than every 1 or 2 weeks. Be sensitive to your body. Sudden increases in intensity can result in injury. Remember: be patient and use common sense. Experiment and find what's right for you.

Trivia...

Sports psychologists believe that there's an important interplay between our personalities and the way in which we work out. They say that the type of person you are affects not only what kind of exercise you like to do, but the way in which you respond to certain forms of exercise. This is why, at the end of a step class, some people feel on a high while others feel like they've been subjected to torture!

How much is too much?

Many people who start an exercise programme make the mistake of trying to progress far too quickly. Over-exercising can be dangerous. Some muscle soreness, or even a "stitch" or cramp is normal, but if you have any of the following symptoms, you should seek medical attention:

- Pains in the chest
- Severe shortness of breath (a little, of course, is expected)
- Dizziness, faintness
- Extreme fatigue
- Feeling sick

The pitfall of most beginners is simply over-exercising.

What if you're on the exercise seesaw?

You need to exercise on a regular basis to develop and maintain physical fitness. You begin to lose fitness progress if you stop exercising for 2 weeks. After 4 to 12 weeks, you lose 50 per cent. You lose 100 per cent of your fitness progress if you stop exercising for 10 to 30 weeks.

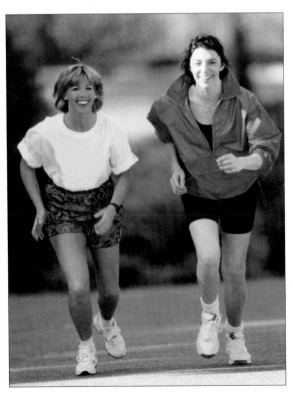

The good news is that it's never too late to start exercising. Recent studies show that 40-year-old women who start walking briskly for half an hour a day, 4 days a week, enjoy almost the same low risk of heart attack as women who have exercised consistently their entire lives.

After engaging in a regular exercise programme for 1 year, your body reacts as if you've been exercising all your life.

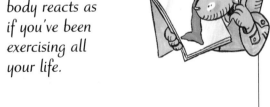

■ **Exercise benefits** *people of all ages – but if you're just starting out, take it slowly and build up your fitness gradually.*

Be accountable

IT'S EXTREMELY HELPFUL to have to be accountable to someone else. *Beginning a fitness programme alone can be difficult because it's so easy to make excuses to yourself. It's much harder to slack off when you have to tell those excuses to someone else.*

Get a partner

Find someone with similar goals – enlist a friend, colleague, family member, or partner – to start with you. Make a plan together, such as walking for half an hour on Monday, Wednesday, and Friday evenings. Or join a class together.

It's important to remember that everyone is different, and each body reacts differently to exercise. Some people will advance to more intense training more rapidly than will others. Somewhere along the way, you may have to change exercise partners so as to keep pace with one another.

Join a class

If you sign up for a class, and pay for it, you are obliged to go. Look around for a convenient class that suits your fitness level.

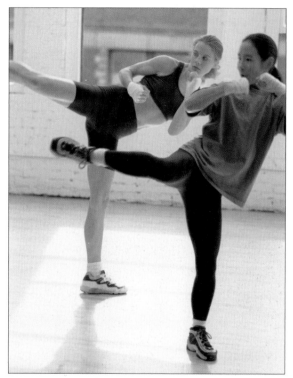

■ **Exercising with a friend** *gives you more motivation to show up to classes because you won't want to let the other person down.*

It doesn't have to be an aerobics class, unless aerobic exercise specifically appeals to you. Just try something that seems like fun. Have you always wanted to tap dance? How about karate?

Don't be afraid to shop around, visit classes, and talk to people to find exactly what you want.

Sign up for a run or walk

There are many walks, runs, and races of various distances happening a few times a year. Many of them are for good causes, such as AIDS and breast cancer research.

I have a friend who has trouble keeping her exercise routine going. Recently, she signed up for a sponsored walk in aid of a cancer charity. She stuck to her walking schedule and increased her speed and distance in the months before. Not only did she get in better shape, she raised £800 for breast cancer research.

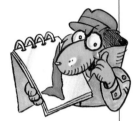

To find an event in your area, check postings at the gym, fitness magazines, and your local paper.

Keep a fitness diary

KEEPING A FITNESS DIARY is an effective way to keep track of your goals and stick to your fitness routine. This can be a plain notebook or diary or an actual "fitness journal" that has lines for weight, goals, calorie counting, and so forth.

What goes into the diary?

To start with, you could note down the results of the fitness assessment given earlier in this chapter. Then, any kind of physical evaluation – one you do at home or a professionally done evaluation – should go into the fitness diary to record your progress.

Write down your short- and long-term goals. You should also log in your workouts right after you do them. You don't have to record only cold, hard facts. If the man ahead of you at the water fountain took too much time and irritated you, write it down and let off steam.

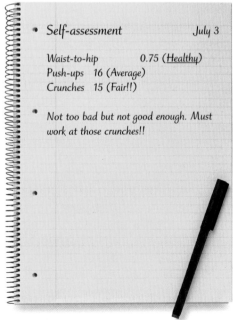

FITNESS DIARY

• Self-assessment   July 3

Waist-to-hip   0.75 (<u>Healthy</u>)
Push-ups   16 (Average)
Crunches   15 (Fair!!)

• Not too bad but not good enough. Must work at those crunches!!

Bring your diary with you everywhere, and write in it every day. If you didn't work out, you could write why you didn't. Some people like to record what they eat. This type of entry helps maintain a balance of calorie intake and expenditure. (To help you monitor progress, at the end of this book you'll find a blank fitness log and exercise diary pages that you can photocopy and fill in.)

What goes in your diary is ultimately up to you, but it should help keep you honest and on track.

Reward yourself

Of course, being fit is its own reward, but to help things along, it's important to recognize when you've reached your goals.

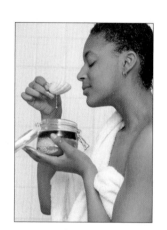

Reward yourself by taking a warm bubble bath, going on a trip to a spa, buying a new outfit, purchasing some new gadget you've had your eye on, having dinner with friends, or even throwing a party.

■ **You deserve a special treat** *when you reach a fitness goal. Why not reward yourself with a bath or shower treatment that will help soothe and relax those aching muscles?*

A simple summary

✓ Assessing your fitness situation is the first step in starting an effective exercise programme.

✓ Recording your weight, flexibility, and muscle strength is an important way to learn what you need to work on.

✓ Setting realistic short- and long-term goals is an effective way to make progress.

✓ Enlisting a partner, joining a class, or signing up for a fitness event makes you accountable to other people. You will be less likely to weasel out of exercise.

✓ An exercise journal helps keep you on track.

✓ Have fun! It's important to reward yourself when you achieve your goals.

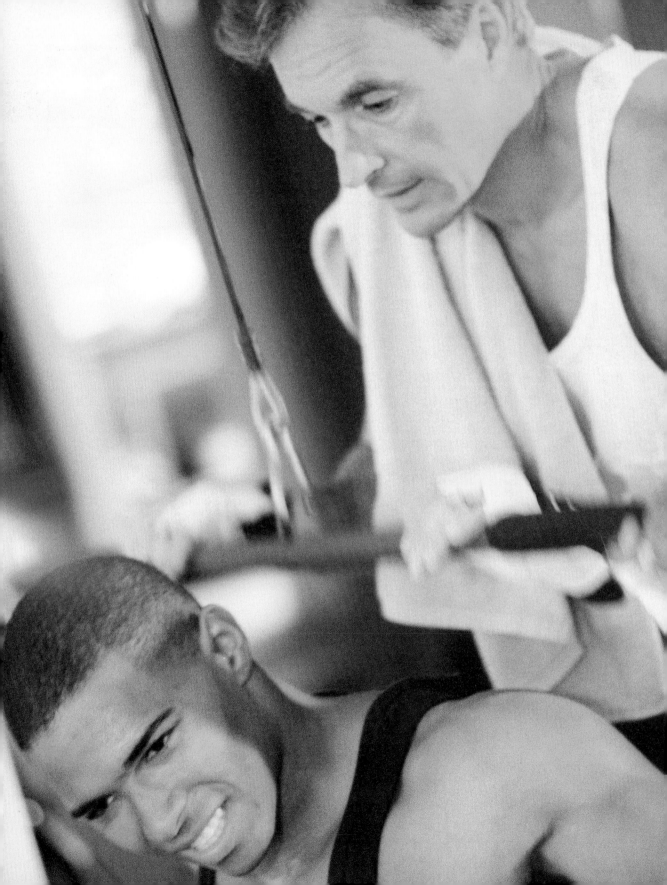

Chapter 3

The Lowdown on Gyms

JOINING A GYM OR HEALTH CLUB is an excellent way to stay in shape, but if the thought of all those complicated-looking machines and toned people in skimpy aerobics outfits makes you want to crawl under the bed, then read on to discover how to find the gym for you.

In this chapter...

✓ Why join a gym?

✓ Finding a gym you like

✓ A simple guide to gym equipment

✓ A rundown on classes

✓ Personal trainers

✓ Gym etiquette

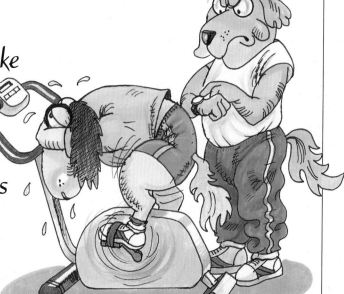

WORKING OUT IN A GYM GIVES YOU A GREATER CHOICE OF EXERCISE AND THE CHANCE TO SOCIALIZE

Why join a gym?

FIRST OF ALL, LET'S DEFINE A GYM. A gym can be a health club, or local leisure centre, or even just a room full of weights. Here, when I talk about gyms, I mean just about any indoor (and sometimes outdoor) facility where people exercise.

What are the benefits of joining a gym or health club? One of the best reasons to join is to take advantage of the variety of activities available. No matter what equipment you have at home, a gym is going to provide more options. The various facilities can help you customize your workout. Let's say you want to build up your shoulders while slimming your chest; it's easier to isolate muscles with the weight machines. More variety also means fewer chances of becoming bored.

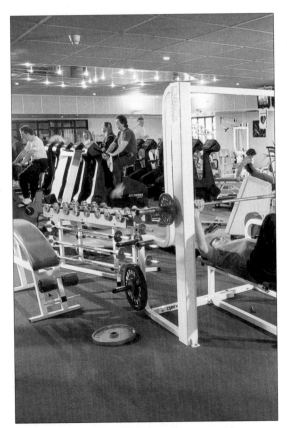

■ **The array of equipment** *at a gym enables you to customize your workout to suit you. It also allows you to vary your routine so you won't get bored.*

Rain, cold, heat, or snow won't cancel your workout. You can work out in any weather (as long as you can get to your gym).

Another reason to go to the gym is to find out what's happening in the local area. Many gyms have announcements for ball games, local sports teams, walks, runs, or other physical activities that might interest you. Some even organize trips, such as skiing holidays. The health club announcement board helps you stay in touch with fitness news and events.

As for making it a habit – joining a gym is a financial commitment. Knowing that you want to get your money's worth might help motivate you to go. If I have a plan to work out at home, I'm more likely to skip it. But if I'm supposed to go to the gym, I treat it like an appointment, and I go. It's like a job that I have to do whether I want to or not, and I'm always glad that I did.

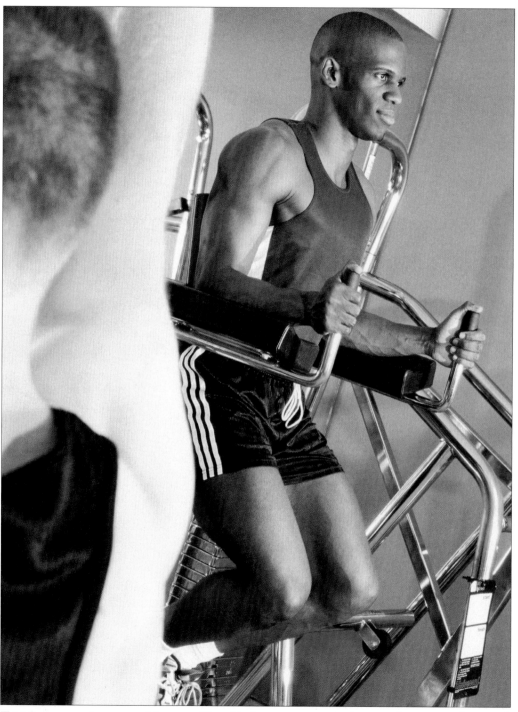

■ **Make an appointment with yourself** *to visit the gym on a regular basis. In this way, you'll get good value from your membership and reap the benefits of increased physical activity.*

Finding a gym you like

THERE ARE ALL KINDS OF GYMS, *but the basic gym will have a fitness room with exercise machines, a free weight (weights that aren't attached to anything) room or area, and a place to stretch – either a stretching room or at least a few mats in the corner. Most also have at least one studio for classes.*

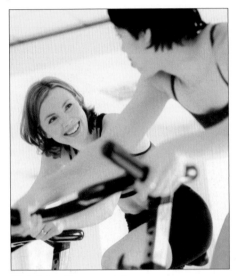

■ **A friendly atmosphere** *at your gym helps to keep you motivated.*

Some have a swimming pool, or squash courts. They all (except single-sex fitness centres) have men's and women's locker rooms or at least changing areas, and some of the fancier gyms have steam rooms, saunas, or Jacuzzis. Some of the higher-end health clubs have juice bars, restaurants, bars, hairdressing salons and beauty treatment rooms, and even a place to drop off your dry cleaning. On the other hand, some gyms are as no-frills as you can get. Some boxing gyms, for example, might have only a ring, some bags, and a few weights.

Walking into a new gym can be intimidating, especially if you don't know where everything is or how to use all the machines. But do be aware that most people are much too busy concentrating on their own workouts to notice you.

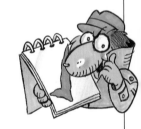

INTERNET

www.gymguide.co.uk

www.goodgymguide.com.au

Find a gym in the UK, or in Australia, by clicking on to one of the above sites.

There are as many types of gyms as there are types of people. Do a little investigating before you take the plunge so you don't end up paying for a membership you never use. Things to consider are location, facilities, and amenities, the clientele, and of course, the price.

Location

There are so many factors to consider when trying to find a gym you want to join. Finding one that's really easy to get to is key. Look for gyms that are near – preferably within walking distance – to your home or work.

Give careful consideration to the facilities and what you like doing. If you love to swim laps, then look for a gym with a pool. Location is still an issue here, though; if you love to swim but there's not a pool within 50 miles, you may have to go with what's available. If you love dance classes, make sure the gym you join offers plenty.

The social scene

Every gym has a different vibe. Some gyms are more social than others, but there is generally a sense of community. Some are like nightclubs, where Lycra-clad men and women mingle and flirt while working out to loud dance music. Others, usually near a corporate area, are places where business deals go down and schmoozing takes place on the squash court. There are a few that are women-only or men-only. Some are no-frills weight rooms where body builders go to pump iron.

My favourites are local community or leisure centre gyms that offer a bit of everything. They are usually friendly and informal and attract local people of all ages. Of course, some people prefer a gym with "extras". At such a gym, patrons get pampered with plush changing facilities, on-site treatment rooms for massages and facials, and a restaurant for post-workout dining. Those are fun, too, but a bit more expensive.

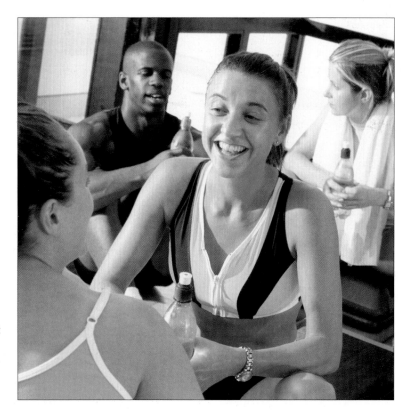

■ **Gyms can be great** *places to meet new people. Classes, in particular, tend to attract a loyal following – so members who turn up regularly soon get to know each other.*

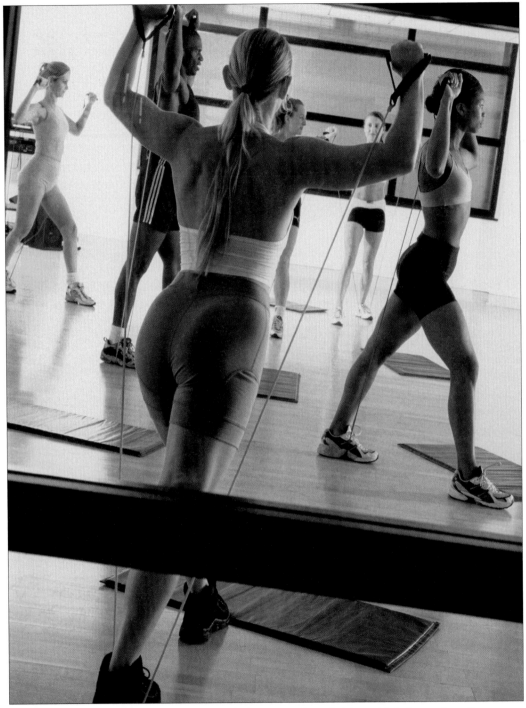

■ **Joining a gym is a big commitment,** *so before you make a decision, visit it first and try the equipment if you can. Going as a guest of a member is a good introduction to the facilities.*

Price

The cost of a membership varies considerably from place to place. If you go to a local authority-run sports centre you can either pay each time you go (up to about £5 per visit), or pay a monthly subscription (typically £25–£40 per month). Fancy health clubs with all the amenities generally charge a joining fee (anything from £50-£500), plus an annual subscription that you can pay up front or in instalments. You can also sign up for 2 or 3 years, but I'd recommend starting off with a 1-year commitment.

Lots of gyms offer special deals – often during January – such as a reduced joining fee, or a lower monthly rate, or, best of all, two for the price of one. Call or visit to find out the prices, as even rates that are posted are subject to change.

Get a free visit

All gyms will let you come for a visit, and many will issue you with a guest pass so that you can sample all that's on offer. Call to book a visit or just turn up and ask if you can have a look around. Look online, too, because sometimes gyms offer day passes on their web sites. Ask friends and colleagues about their gyms. If you know anyone who belongs to a gym you're interested in, ask if you can be his or her guest for a day.

Most gyms allow guests for free or for a small charge. An added benefit in joining a gym where you know someone is that you'll have a workout partner. If you're not sure about a gym, try to visit it at the times you're likely to go there. If you're going to go at lunchtime, visit then. Or if you'll try to sneak in early exercise before work, visit in the early morning. Gyms can have a different atmosphere depending on the time of day. Most places are crowded in the early morning and in the evening.

The best way to find a gym you like is to visit.

Questions to ask before joining

Once you've found a gym you like, and before signing on the dotted line, ask what's included. If you've selected a gym because you love the classes they offer, but find out that classes cost extra, then you might want to consider paying class-by-class at a non-member rate. Or, if it's the squash court you're interested in, but you find out that the cost of hiring a court is too expensive, then you may want to keep looking. But don't get discouraged too quickly.

If there's only one gym you can get to, then try and find something you like there. Some gyms also offer a free session with a personal trainer. Ask questions and make sure you get all the perks that you're entitled to.

A simple guide to gym equipment

MOST GYMS DIVIDE EXERCISE MACHINES into categories based on the type of exercise they provide – cardio, strength training, and stretching. Although health clubs usually give you an induction session (ask for it if it's not offered), it's good to know what to expect. Most equipment is designed to imitate some activity such as running, biking, or rowing, but in a climate-controlled environment. Most have manual or programmed settings, so you can make your session on the machine as challenging or as easy as you like. Take it easy when you're first getting a feel for the machines, and work up to a higher intensity. Also, experiment – play with the settings and find out what works best for you.

Many of these machines are similar to those you could stock in your home gym, but commercial equipment is a bit sturdier. Following is a rundown of equipment you're likely to find and how to use it.

Elliptical crosstrainer

Introduced in 1995, the elliptical crosstrainer is one of the newest kids on the block, and now it's one of the most popular forms of exercise in the health clubs. By using this machine, you can burn as many calories as if you were out jogging, but with less

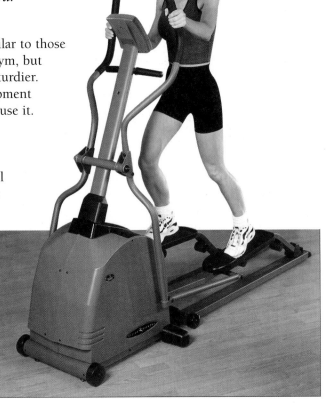

■ **Crosstrainers** *are designed to alleviate strain on joints. Those with moveable handlebars work both the upper and lower body.*

stress on the joints and less perceived physical exertion. This means that it feels a little easier than running. Working out on the elliptical crosstrainer is a good exercise for building lower-body muscle groups.

Using the elliptical crosstrainer

In a standing position, put your feet on the pedals (like a stair climber). As you pedal, your feet move in an elliptical orbit. You can adjust the size of the orbit and the resistance level. You can also choose to go forward or backward. Many elliptical crosstrainers come with moveable handlebars to give you an upper body workout too and to burn more calories.

Treadmill

A treadmill looks a bit like a conveyor belt large enough for one person. Treadmills are designed to give you a good cardio workout by walking or running. This is an excellent way to get in a jog or walk on a rainy day or if you don't want to travel too far. Some distance runners with knee injuries prefer to train on the treadmill instead of outside so that they're not miles away from home if they have to stop. Most health clubs have at least two treadmills.

Using the treadmill

You can adjust the belt to any speed, from slow walking to sprinting. Start slowly to get the feel of walking on a treadmill; it takes a little getting used to. Once you get a feel for it, you can adjust the gradient to make it feel as if you're walking on a flat surface or going up or

■ **Treadmills** *give you a good cardiovascular workout. You can walk or jog at your own pace and at your chosen gradient.*

down hills. There are handles under the console, or at the sides if you need them, but don't hang on while you're working out. The handles are for getting your balance when starting and stopping. When using a treadmill, run or walk as if you were outside. That means keep your back straight and let your arms move freely by your side.

Never lean over on the handlebars or consoles of exercise equipment – they're not there to support you throughout the exercise. The only time you can lean over the handlebars is when you're standing up because you're on a steep incline on a stationary bike.

Treadmills come with an automatic warm-up and cool-down, which means that they start and stop gradually. Even if you want to go fast, you don't have to worry about the belt suddenly speeding up or abruptly stopping. If you're in the middle of a timed workout and you want to stop, don't panic: you can press the bright red stop button at any time. The belt will slow down, and you can step off on either side. If you find you can't keep up and you're moving backwards during the workout, then you should slow the pace a bit.

Stationary bicycle

Stationary bikes can provide a very challenging workout. Upright bikes look and feel much like regular bikes. **Recumbent** bikes are the kind you pedal with your feet out in front rather than down.

> **DEFINITION**
>
> **Recumbent** *means reclining, so whenever you see a recumbent bike or a recumbent stair climber, you know that means the exercise is done in a seated position with legs out in front (instead of below). This position is good for people with lower back trouble because the back is supported.*

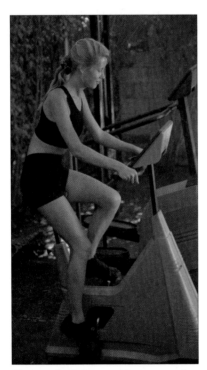

■ **Upright bikes** *enable you to cycle on the flat or up and down hills as if riding a regular bike. Remember to adjust the height of your seat before you start pedalling.*

Using the upright or recumbent bike

Adjust the seat when you get on so that your knee is almost straight when you pedal all the way down. If your seat is too high (or too far back on the recumbent bike), you'll over-extend your knee. If your seat is too low (or too close), your knees will be bent, and your knees and hips won't get a full range of motion. You can adjust the resistance level to make it feel as if you're going up or down hills, but the speed is dictated by how fast you pedal. Remember, don't lean over the handlebars (unless you're standing up on the upright bike) and grip them lightly.

Many cardio machines come with the options of setting the amount of time you want to exercise, the distance, incline (or resistance level), and speed. Many can also measure how many calories you've burned and measure your heart rate.

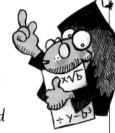

Be wary of calories burned and heart rate as measured by cardio machines, because they're not always right. If you lean on the handlebars, for example, you're not burning as many calories as the machine says you are.

Stair climber

Also called stairstepper or stepper, this machine works your lower body because it feels just like climbing stairs. The pedals adjust to various resistance levels.

Using the stair climber

Put your feet on the pedals and move them as if you were climbing stairs. Stand up straight and, as always, don't lean over the rails. You can adjust the intensity of the workout. If you take bigger steps, you work the buttocks more; smaller steps work the legs and calves.

Rowing machine

This low-to-the-ground apparatus is designed to give you a good upper body workout by mimicking the motion of rowing a boat.

Using the rowing machine

Adjust the seat so your feet are securely on the foot boards when you're leaning back. Begin pushing back with your legs before you begin pulling on the handles. Keep your elbows in by your sides and pull on the oars. Return to the starting position in one fluid motion and repeat.

■ **Rowing machines** *are designed to work the upper body and build cardiovascular strength.*

Trivia...

While some people enjoy zoning out to the repetitive motion of exercising on machines, others get bored. Many gyms have TVs on the wall so you can watch while you work. Some have headphone sets on machine consoles that allow you to tune into a TV channel or radio station. In the US, many gym-goers are now able to listen to CDs or surf the Web while they sweat. Could be coming to a gym near you soon!

Weight machines

These are machines that provide an alternative to lifting free weights. A major benefit of using the weight machines is that they're safer because the weight stacks are held by pulleys and cables locked into a track.

So, if you can no longer lift the load, or if you have to stop for some reason, the weights aren't going to come crashing down. Also, machines offer better muscle isolation. They're usually grouped together to make a multi-station full-body muscle-building workout. In fact, just by moving a cable or pulling a pin, you can perform as many as 70 different weight routines on some multi-station machines.

The great user-friendly aspect of these machines is that there's usually an explanation and diagram of the area of the body worked during the exercise, plus a detailed explanation on how to do the motion properly. If you've never used the weight machine you're facing, be sure to read the directions carefully. Each machine is a bit different.

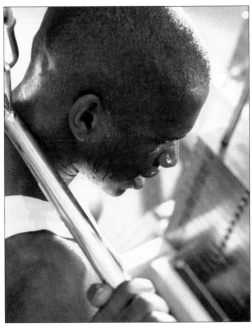

■ **Weight machines** *provide an effective and safe way of strengthening and toning the muscles.*

On Cybex machines (a brand that's used in many gyms), step-by-step directions are written out with a diagram that shows positioning, movement, and primary and secondary muscles trained.

Using the weight machines

First, adjust the seat and handles (the parts that you adjust vary from machine to machine) so that you will lift with proper form. Keep in mind where your pivot point is – this is explained in the directions on the machine. If you're lifting weight with your arm, for example, make sure that your elbow is where it's supposed to be. Next, select the amount of weight you wish to lift, usually by moving the pin to the corresponding weight. Start with lighter weight and work your way up.

As you perform the motion, it is important that you do not let the machines do all the work for you. This means, not letting velocity help you along. These lifts should be done slowly, with the lifting and recovery done with care. Most lifts can be done by lifting on a count of two and returning on a count of four.

A rundown on classes

THERE'S MORE THAN ONE WAY TO SHAKE, shimmy, or pump your way to being fit. These days, there's an exercise class for everyone's taste. I really enjoy them because I usually work out for longer when I'm in a class; I get restless going round and round on a treadmill. Plus, classes can teach you new moves that you can incorporate into your regular workout, and you can meet new friends (if you want to).

What's best for you?

Sometimes, I'm so busy trying to follow the directions that I don't even realize I'm sweating. Remember, you can always adapt each class to your level. If it's your first time, it's okay if you don't do each move exactly right. (It's also okay if you want to hang out near the back and watch the first few times.) Here's a simple description of classes to help you find what's best for you.

Trivia...

US fitness guru and Reebok master trainer, Gin Miller, created step aerobics in 1989. Now step training is offered in 97 per cent of health clubs in the United Kingdom and abroad. For more info about Gin, go to www.ginmiller.com.

Aerobics

The most popular kind of fitness class since the '70s, aerobics classes include movements that get you sweating and breathing heavily and that raise your heart rate. A class called simply "aerobics" will be like a high-energy dance class. Traditional aerobics classes are broken up into categories: low-impact, high-impact, and high/low. Low-impact is good for beginners or for people who are overweight. One foot always stays in contact with the floor, but low-impact still gets your heart rate up. High-impact is a little harder on your joints because there's a lot of hopping and jumping. High/low combo, as the name suggests, is a combination of the two.

Kickboxing, spinning, step, and many other classes fall under the aerobics category because they get your heart rate up, but they are usually listed separately.

Kickboxing

This newly popular class incorporates martial arts moves in a high-energy workout. Lots of front, side, and back kicks are combined with jab, cross, and hook punches. It's a great way to get out some aggression. You learn some good moves, but it's not a self-defence class because you're punching and kicking in time to the music.

Step

In this action-packed aerobics class, you step up and down on adjustable platforms. These classes involve following a set of maneouvres that can get quite complicated.

Studio cycling

In these group classes, an instructor guides you through an intense cycling journey on stationary bikes. These classes are usually high intensity, with loud house music pumping while you pedal at different speeds at various inclines.

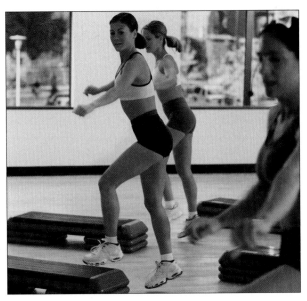

HIGH-IMPACT STEP CLASS

Sculpting or "power" sculpting

If you see the word "sculpting", prepare to lift weights or do other weight-bearing exercise such as push-ups and crunches. The aim is to build muscle and "sculpt" your physique.

Boot camp

This is a no-frills class that's modelled on military training. The instructor usually barks orders for the classic exercises like jumping jacks, push-ups, sit-ups, and squats. This one is more popular with men.

"Abs" classes

These refer to classes full of moves to work everyone's favourite spot – the *abdominal muscles*. That means lots of crunches, sit-ups, and other lower body exercises.

DEFINITION

Abdominal muscles *are the group of muscles that run along the front and side of your trunk.*

Mind/body

These days, most gyms offer a variety of "mind-body" classes. These classes usually include a lot of stretching, conscious breathing, and being mindful of your body. Some of the more popular ones are yoga and Pilates, which we'll delve into in Chapter 9. Also popular are the Feldenkrais Method and the Alexander Technique, both designed to enhance physical activity by bringing awareness to your body.

Personal trainers

PERSONAL TRAINERS ARE HIRED FITNESS coaches who can assess your fitness situation and get you going on the right track by working with you one-on-one. They can help custom design your workout, choose the equipment that's right for you, and guide you through the moves safely and effectively. Some gyms will offer one free session when you join. If yours does, by all means take advantage of it.

Some personal trainers are on staff at gyms; other trainers work on a freelance basis. If you can't find a personal trainer at your gym, check the noticeboard or buy a magazine about fitness and look through the small ads. When looking for a personal trainer, find one who has been certified by a legitimate fitness group or who has a degree in physical education. Most charge by the hour, and the prices can range from £20 to £75.

One of the perks of having a personal trainer is that if you have an appointment with one, it's going to be harder to get out of exercising than if you were going to the gym by yourself.

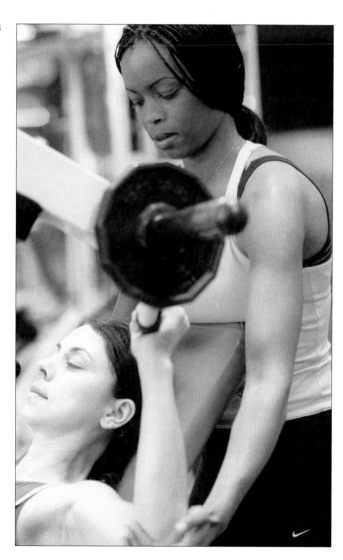

■ **A personal trainer** *can be a great help, particularly at the start of a fitness campaign when you may need to be shown how to make the correct moves.*

Gym etiquette

MOST GYMS HAVE SIGNS about rules and behaviour, but here are some general rules about gym conduct that can save you from getting a growl or two from frustrated fellow exercisers. Much of the following is common sense, but there may be some things that you wouldn't necessarily think of unless you were already a gym aficionado.

Some machines, like treadmills, bikes, and cross trainers, have sign-up sheets. If the gym is crowded, look for a sign-up sheet before hopping onto a recently vacated machine. Here are a few more etiquette points to remember:

1. Don't be a machine hog. When it's crowded or when people are waiting, don't stay on any piece of equipment for more than 20 minutes. Look for a sign – some gyms have specific time limits

2. Don't hover over someone when you're waiting for a machine

3. "Work in" with someone. This means taking it in turns to work out on a piece of equipment – usually the weight machines

4. Don't leave sweat on the machines (or anywhere). Wipe machines or mats with a towel or tissue paper after using them

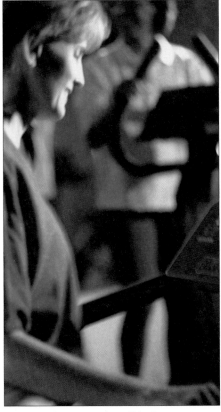

■ **At peak times,** *there'll be heavy demand for the machines, so don't take more than your fair share of time.*

5. Don't fill up your water bottle at the fountain when there are people waiting

6. On the running track: slower runners stay on the inside of the track. Also, don't stop suddenly to check your heart or tie your shoe because there might be someone right behind you

7. In the pool: share the lane. If there are two people sharing a lane, stay on one side. If there are more than two, swim in circles, always staying on the right

8 Sauna/steam room: in single-sex sauna and steam rooms, you can wear a towel or be nude. In shared ones, wear swimming gear

9 Showers and changing: some gyms have shared showers; others have individual ones. There are usually areas separated by curtains you can change clothes behind if you're shy

10 Massage: depending on the gym, you can either be nude or wear a swimming costume or trunks when getting a massage. If you're not sure, ask someone

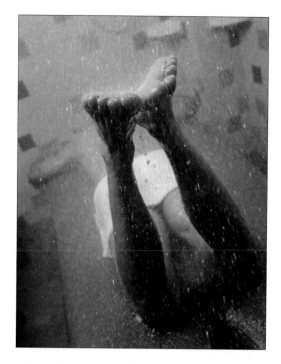

■ **A towel is** *all you're likely to need in a single sex steam room, but if in doubt, ask.*

A simple summary

✔ Joining a gym is an excellent way to enhance your commitment to exercise.

✔ Knowing what you're going to find at the gym can make the process a whole lot easier.

✔ It's important to find a gym that's convenient and in your price range – and that has activities and people you like.

✔ There is a wide-range of exercise equipment that can help you reach your fitness goals.

✔ Exercise classes aren't just aerobics and leg warmers any more.

✔ Personal trainers can help you custom design a fitness plan.

✔ There is a code of conduct in the gym.

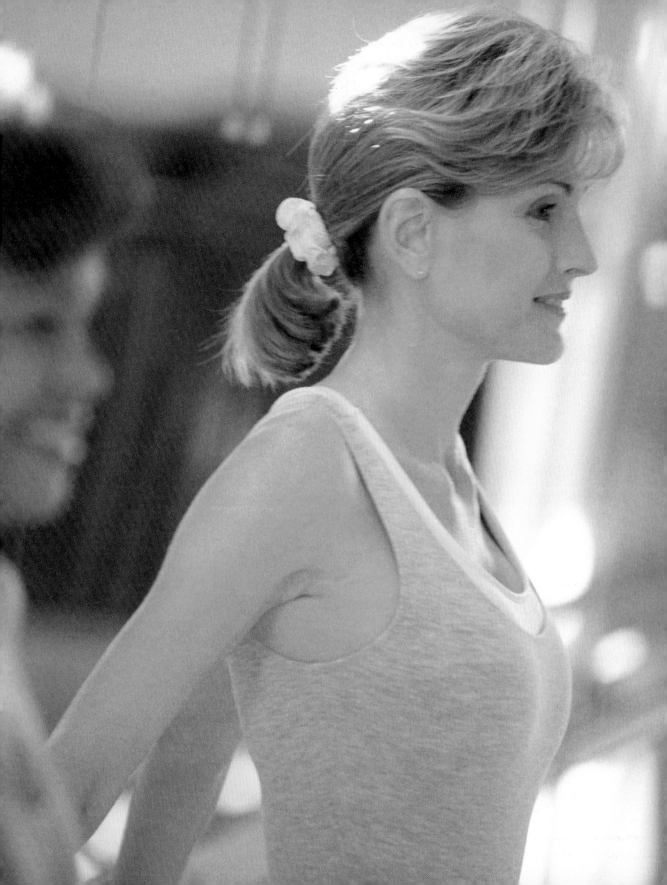

Chapter 4

Simple Fitness Tools

READY TO HIT THE GYM? Forget anything? Check out all the things you'll need from a well-packed gym bag to a fun and functional fitness wardrobe. We'll talk about fabrics that'll keep you dry and comfortable to make your workout more enjoyable. We'll help you find a shoe that fits well so as to save your feet from unnecessary aches and pains. Step up your workout with a heart-rate monitor, pedometer, or even a personal stereo. Finally, read about gears and gadgets with all the bells and whistles to turn you into a pro. Read on!

In this chapter...

✓ Gym bag essentials

✓ Sweating in style and comfort

✓ If the shoe fits...

✓ Simple fitness gear and gadgets

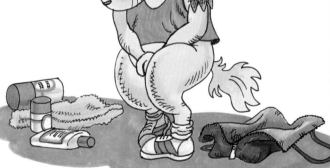

THE RIGHT CLOTHES, SHOES, AND ACCESSORIES WILL HELP YOU WIN THE FITNESS BATTLE

Gym bag essentials

HAVING THE RIGHT ACCOUTREMENTS *can help you rise to any occasion, especially exercise. Are you going to stop running just after you've bought a new pair of running shoes? No! Nor would you bail out on your fitness routine once you have the necessities. But what are they?*

Although many things that go in the gym bag may seem obvious, there are plenty of items you might not think of until you're there, and it's too late. You don't want to have to cut your workout short or leave the changing room in only a towel because you forgot something.

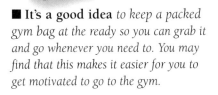

Checklist

Here's a list of gym bag items to help you prepare for working out in style and comfort:

■ **It's a good idea** *to keep a packed gym bag at the ready so you can grab it and go whenever you need to. You may find that this makes it easier for you to get motivated to go to the gym.*

1. **A towel or two**: in addition to the towel you will need for your post-workout shower, bring a small towel to wipe the sweat – yours as well as that of the sweathog before you – off the machines. It's not only courteous, it's the rule in some gyms. Bring another, larger towel to dry off after a shower or steam. Some gyms offer towels free or for a small fee. These are usually good for wiping the sweat off machines, but are often a bit too small to wrap up in after working out. Bring your own back-up towel just in case, especially if it's your first time to a gym

2. **Coins for lockers**: most gyms don't allow you to bring your coat or bags into the workout room. Even if they do permit it, it's a good idea to lock belongings in a locker so you don't have to worry about keeping an eye on them, and they won't get in the way. All gyms have lockers for you to put your extra things in. You may need to insert a coin (usually £1) to release the locker key. When you've finished with the locker for that session, you get the coin back.

Don't know where to put that key while you work out? Tie it to your shoelaces. Unlace through one eyelet and slide the key onto the shoelace, re-thread it, and tie. Make sure your key is steady and won't scrape up against your other leg or fall off.

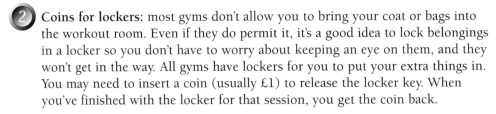

You are usually only allowed to use a locker for the duration of your gym visit, so don't leave any gear behind – even overnight – because you could return to find that it has been removed. If you want to keep stuff at the gym, you may be able to hire your own personal locker for an annual or monthly fee

3. **Shower shoes:** a pair of waterproof sandals that you can wear into the shower and around the pool can save you from having to go barefoot. Bacteria, such as the kind that cause athlete's foot, tend to lurk around warm moist places like gym shower floors. I sometimes forget my sandals and end up getting my running shoes wet when I try to tiptoe into the shower without going barefoot. Most department stores sell shower shoes – but they don't need to be expensive. You can find a pair of lightweight shoes on the high street for a few pounds

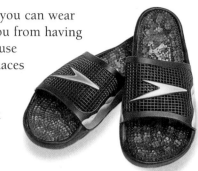

SHOWER SHOES

4. **Plastic bag:** an extra plastic bag comes in handy to put your workout clothes and wet towel in when you're done. Without one, you risk getting everything else in your bag damp

5. **Toiletries:** if you're going to shower at the gym, don't forget shampoo, soap, lotion, and deodorant. (This is especially necessary if you hit the gym on a lunch break and have to go back to work.) Some higher-end gyms have toiletries such as deodorant, lotion, soap, and even hairspray in the changing room. Keeping some grooming and shower items that you like in your gym bag may help motivate you to go

6. **Hair band:** bring something to keep your hair out of the way. If you have long hair, tuck a few extra rubber bands or clips in your bag

7. **Hat or headband:** these can help keep the sweat from dripping into your eyes while you're working out hard. If you have short hair, this is also a good way of keeping it out of the way

TOILETRIES

8. **Sweatbands:** sweatbands or wristbands help keep your hands dry if you're lifting weights or playing a racquet sport

9. **Water bottle:** staying hydrated is especially important when you're exercising. Bring a durable bottle of water to drink from during or after your workout. Many gyms don't allow open containers, but a water bottle is permitted in the workout area

10 **Snack:** throw a piece of fruit or an energy bar in your bag for the post-workout munchies. This way you won't end up buying junk food

11 **Clothing options:** keep a short-sleeved T-shirt and a tank top, shorts, and sweat pants in your bag, because you never know how cold or warm it's going to be in the gym

12 **Extra socks and underwear:** it's no fun having to wear the damp socks or underwear you worked out in home from the gym. Bring extra pairs to change into post-exercise

13 **Fitness diary:** keep your fitness diary in your bag so you can check up on your progress beforehand and update it immediately afterwards. If you're recording specifics like how much weight you lifted or how far you ran, you might want to bring it into the gym with you

■ **A fitness diary** *is a compulsory item for anyone who is serious about getting fit.*

MOBILE FIRST AID KIT

a **Pain reliever:** toss in a bottle of aspirin or paracetamol for aches and soreness

b **Plasters:** keep a few plasters in assorted sizes in your gym bag – they can ease the pain of a new blister

c **Sun block:** if your workout takes you outside, protect your skin with waterproof and sweat-proof sun block

d **Feminine protection for surprises:** tampons are small and discreet. Panty liners are a good option for the between days or for extra protection while working out

Sports-specific items

Of course, each sport demands specific equipment, such as a racquet for tennis, but here are some necessities for other gym-related activities.

For lifting weights

1. **Weight-lifting gloves**: lifting weights without gloves can hurt and can make your palms calloused and rough. Gloves give you a better grip, which can make hoisting kilos (or pounds) a bit easier

2. **Weight belt**: a weight belt adds back support and can prevent injury and improve your form

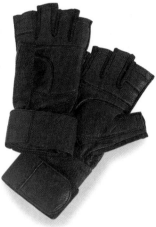

GLOVES WITH WRIST SUPPORT

Trivia...

Swimming costumes in the 1800s were large and cumbersome and were made out of heavy materials such as wool or flannel. In addition, some women went so far as sewing lead weights into the hems of their "bathing gowns" to keep the dresses from floating up and exposing their legs. Imagine swimming laps in those!

For swimming

1. **Swimming costume or trunks**: these should be comfortable and stay on securely. Nylon and nylon/Lycra blends are good fabrics

2. **Swimming cap**: many pools require every swimmer to wear a swimming cap. Rubber caps are inexpensive, and some gyms sell these. Cloth caps are easier to put on and don't stick to your hair when being removed. If you have long hair and are not wearing a cap, make sure you tie your hair back and out of the way

3. **Goggles**: the most important thing to look for in goggles is a good fit. When trying them on, make sure the eye pieces fit securely by checking the suction action before you put the strap on. You can get goggles with special features such as anti-fog or UV sun protection.

If you can't see much without your glasses, like me, wear your contacts and a good pair of goggles when swimming laps. It's easier than trying to find a safe place to put glasses within reach by the pool or bumping into people underwater

INTERNET

www.speedo.com

Click here for info on Speedo goggles.

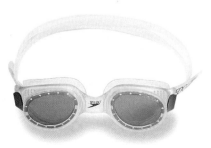

SWIMMING GOGGLES

Sweating in style and comfort

NO GYM BAG WOULD BE COMPLETE *without clothes. But what do you need besides a T-shirt? Of course, you can work out in almost anything. I saw a woman at my gym the other day running on the treadmill in her torn long underwear. I'm sure it worked fine, but she might've been a little more comfortable in a pair of sweat pants.*

Having fun new workout clothes can help get you in the mood. Even when I work out at home, I find that I put more into my workout in my workout clothes than when I just exercise in my pyjamas. (Hey, I'm at home. Who's looking, right?) Putting on my workout clothes is a way of dedicating that time to exercise time. It's like a uniform. Plus, it doesn't hurt to find workout clothes you like and that make you feel good. If you're at the gym in rags, your self-confidence might take a plunge. It's added incentive to work out if you have some comfortable and alluring new clothes.

The most important thing to look for in workout clothes is comfort and mobility. You want clothes that you don't have to think about too much or tug into place every minute.

A T-shirt and shorts are fine to get you started. Don't let not having the right outfit stop you from working out.

In choosing exercise clothes, you must consider what you're going to be doing – what activity and in what environment. If you're about to embark upon a mountain-biking regimen, your needs will be different than if you've signed up for a kickboxing class, for example. Also, are you going to be mostly inside or outside? Is it going to be cold or hot?

Cold weather tips

DEFINITION

Moisture wicking *material helps remove excess moisture from your body.*

Wearing layers is the key to staying comfortable when your workout takes you outside in cold weather. Against your skin, wear *moisture wicking* material, or fabric that allows your skin to breathe. Then add extra layers depending on how cold it's going to be. Add middle layers such as fleece or wool and top it off with a wind-resistant jacket or coat. Keep your extremities covered with a hat and gloves or mittens.

Hot weather tips

To stay cool, wear loose, breathable clothing. Light colours are best if you're going to be in the sun. Light colours reflect sun while dark colours absorb it and make you warmer.

Keep in mind that 100 per cent cotton clothing doesn't dry as well as some synthetic moisture-wicking materials. If you're going on an outdoor adventure, avoid 100 per cent cotton clothes because they tend to get wet and stay wet. If it's a short workout in the gym you're doing, then cotton is fine. I still like cotton because it's so soft and comfortable.

Shopping list

Here is a good shopping list for fitness wear:

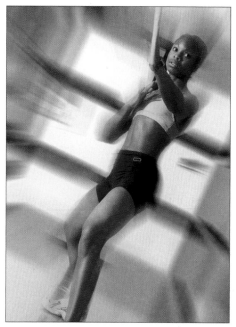

- **Shorts:** a comfy non-chafing pair of shorts belongs in any gym wardrobe. Make sure you have full range of motion, without revealing anything. Shorts with a wide hem at the bottom tend to stay put a bit better
- **T-shirts:** have at least a couple of T-shirts on hand. They're cheap and comfortable
- **Tank tops:** these shirts are great for days when the gym is hot. Plus, tank tops free your arms up, and you can check out your form while you work out
- **Sweatshirt:** a sweatshirt is an easy item to throw on if you're cold, especially after a workout when you're damp from sweating
- **Tracksuit:** these can come in handy to wear over other workout clothes, to get you to the gym and back. Or, wear them in the gym while you exercise. Tracksuits come in all styles and price ranges – think about what you need it for before purchasing

■ **Buying stylish** *new workout gear can really motivate you to get to the gym – if only because it gives you the opportunity to wear it.*

- **Socks:** get socks that don't bunch up around the toe or creep down at the back. You also want to make sure they aren't constricting and that they don't leave a mark on your ankles or calves. It's worth spending a bit more for well-cushioned, high-quality socks that can add a little spring to your step
- **Sports bras and athletic supporters:** these are necessary items if you're running or doing aerobics or basically any time you're going to be jumping or bouncing a lot. There are many different styles to choose from. Look for brands that offer good support and comfort

Now you are armed and ready to hit the gym with style. Posing and grunting are optional.

If the shoe fits …

THE RIGHT SHOE CAN MAKE *all the difference to your workout. There are as many different kinds of exercise shoes as there are people to wear them, but here are some simple facts to help you find the shoe for you.*

For basic fitness, cross trainers and running shoes are the most popular. Cross training is a combination of exercises – a mix of aerobics and strength training, for example. Cross trainers are shoes that are designed to handle a variety of workouts. Cross trainers are good for workouts in which the foot movements are mostly lateral such as in aerobics, step classes, racquet sports, or dancing.

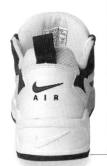

CROSS TRAINERS

Running shoes are great for foot movements that are up and down, such as when running, jogging, walking, or doing a combination of any of these. Running shoes are also good for stair climbing, stationary biking, or even weight training.

Other than that, many sports require specific shoes. Among these are biking, rock climbing, and dance such as ballet or tap.

Know your feet

In order to find the best shoe for you, it's important to get to know your feet. Beyond knowing if your feet are wide or narrow, knowing what kind of arch you have can help you find the shoe that fits. Take the arch test on the next page to find out if you have a high, low, or medium arch.

If you have a low arch, you probably tend to over-**pronate**, which means that you land on the inside of your foot. Look for shoes that are stiff and firm so they control excess motion.

This area would show wear if you over-pronate

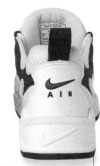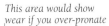

This area would show wear if you under-pronate

■ **Check whether you** *over-pronate or under-pronate before buying new shoes. If either applies, it's important to choose shoes that will best suit your type of feet.*

> **DEFINITION**
>
> *To* **pronate** *is to turn or rotate the sole of the foot so that the inner edge of the sole bears the body's weight.*

THE ARCH TEST

Lay a piece of dark paper flat on the floor (not on carpet). Get your foot wet and take a step on the paper. Or step on a dark towel and leave a footprint when you get out of the shower. Take a look at your footprint and compare it with the ones below.

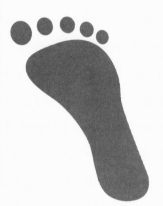

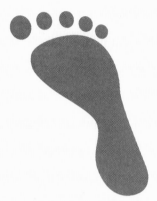

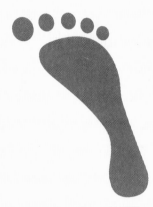

1 **Low arch**

A full foot image indicates a low, flexible arch. Also known as a flat foot, this foot type tends to over-pronate.

2 **Medium arch**

An in-between image shows a medium, neutral arch. This is the most common type of foot.

3 **High arch**

A curvy, incomplete image reveals a high, rigid arch. This type of foot, which is rare, tends to under-pronate and doesn't absorb shock very well.

If you have a high arch, you're probably under-pronating, which is landing on the outside of your foot. Look for shoes that are cushioned and have a firm heel and flexible forefoot.

A medium arch is neutral. People with medium arches should look for shoes that are soft and flexible.

Now that you know what kind of foot you have, you can ask questions about different brands and makes when you go shoe shopping. Shop around to find the brand that is a good fit for your particular feet. The brand of running shoes that fits your best friend perfectly might not fit you so well.

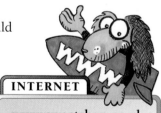

INTERNET

www.sweatshop.co.uk

Visit this site to find out about running shoes, and get running tips and links.

Simple fitness gear and gadgets

THERE ARE PLENTY *of exercise gadgets out there, some useful and others not. Here is a list of items that could come in handy.*

Don't get swept up and buy a wardrobe full of gadgets you don't need. Before you buy high-quality running shoes, tracksuit, or other expensive equipment make sure you enjoy running.

Heart-rate monitors

Although you can measure your heart rate with just your finger and a watch, heart-rate monitors allow you to get an accurate reading of your heart rate without having to stop exercising. Heart-rate monitors have become very easy to use. With a press of a button you can keep track of your heart rate while you exercise. Many also come with features designed to help you with other exercise goals. Some count calories or have an alarm that sounds when you haven't worked out in 3 days. Others have watch, alarm, stopwatch, and calendar functions. There are many different styles and brands of monitors on the market from the basic to multi-featured high-tech models.

Most heart-rate monitors come with a chest strap that measures the signal from your heart and transmits it to a wrist-worn heart-rate monitor that displays the heart rate and any other information. Some of the newest models are worn as watches, with no chest strap. Heart-rate monitors cost anything from £20 to £175.

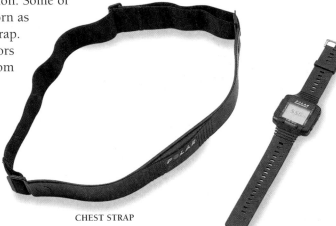

CHEST STRAP

HEART-RATE MONITOR

INTERNET

www.cardiosport.com

www.sarkproducts.com

UK-based Cardiosport offers heart-rate monitors to suit every need, while the US Sark Products site features Cardiosport and Polar ranges.

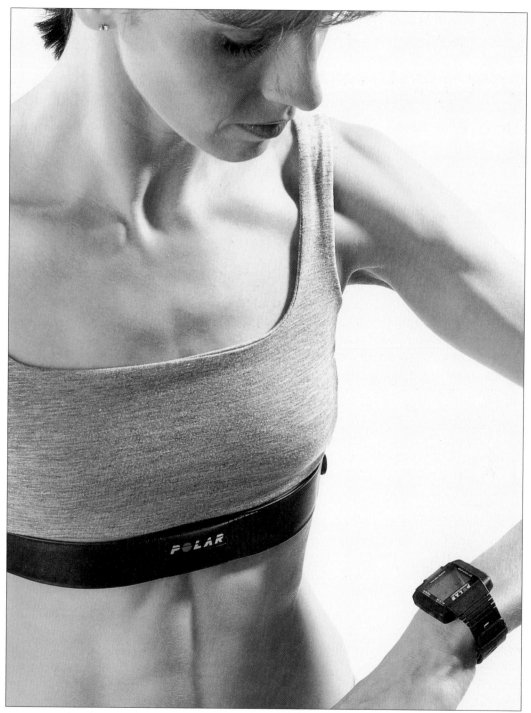

■ **A heart-rate monitor** *makes it easy to keep checking your heart as you exercise. Many models also feature a calorie counter, stopwatch, alarm, and other functions.*

Personal stereos

Since it's not very convenient to drag your stereo equipment to the gym, personal stereos are the best way to listen to music while working out. Music can enhance your exercise experience. It can add a little spice to your workout. It's more fun pedalling on the stationary bike or running on the treadmill to the beat of your favourite song.

Some gyms take music extremely seriously and play music throughout. But if your gym doesn't, or if you don't particularly like what's being played, you may prefer to create your own workout soundtrack and listen to it on your personal stereo.

INTERNET

www.sony.com

www.philips.co.uk

SONY is the manufacturer of the original Walkman, and still makes every kind of personal stereo. Another high-tech personal stereo is the tiny Philips Rush Digital Audio Player MP3.

There are all kinds of personal stereos, from the basic SONY Walkman radio player to a tiny MP3 player that clips on to your waistband.

When looking for a personal stereo to use while working out, there are a few things to keep in mind: make sure the headphones won't slip off your head while you work out; make sure the body of the stereo is small and portable and can clip on to your waistband (or somewhere) without falling off; and beware of cords that can get tangled up.

Here's a tip for you multi-taskers: with your own portable equipment, you can catch up with the radio news or listen to talk shows, or even listen to books on tape.

■ **Listening to a personal stereo** *while exercising can make a workout more enjoyable. Many people find that running to the rhythm of an upbeat song helps spur them on.*

Pedometers

Pedometers measure how far you've walked or run by counting steps taken. Step counting can be a good way to bump up your exercise programme a few notches. If you want to add a few more steps to your day, for example, measure how far you go in your daily tasks. If you wear a pedometer all day and watch the count, you may choose to walk a little further. Also, you can see how far your favourite walking route is. If you have no idea how far your favourite walk is, follow the route with a pedometer and get the facts.

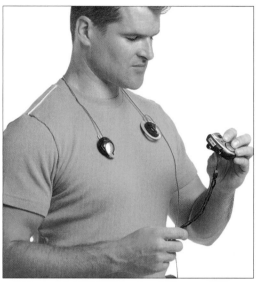

■ **Using a pedometer** *is a good way to bump up your exercise programme. This easy-to-use tool counts the number of steps you have walked or run in a day – or an exercise session – so you can set yourself targets to increase them.*

To use a pedometer, you have to input your stride. Although most come with detailed instructions, you can easily calculate your stride by measuring a 3-metre (10-foot) length on the sidewalk. Walk the 3 metres (10 ft), walking naturally, and count the number of steps. Divide 3 by the number of steps you took to cover the distance. If you took four steps, for example, divide 3 by 4 to yield 0.75 metres (2.5 ft); that's your stride length. To work out your stride length in feet, simply divide 10 by the number of steps you took.

Pedometers are small and easy to use. Most cost between £12 and £50. Some of the more expensive models come with extras such as a stopwatch or calorie counter.

A simple summary

✔ Make a list and check it twice. Keeping a gym bag packed and ready makes it easy to get moving.

✔ The right exercise clothes can improve the quality of your workout.

✔ Knowing your foot can help you find the perfect exercise shoe.

✔ Heart-rate monitors, pedometers, and personal stereos are great workout aids.

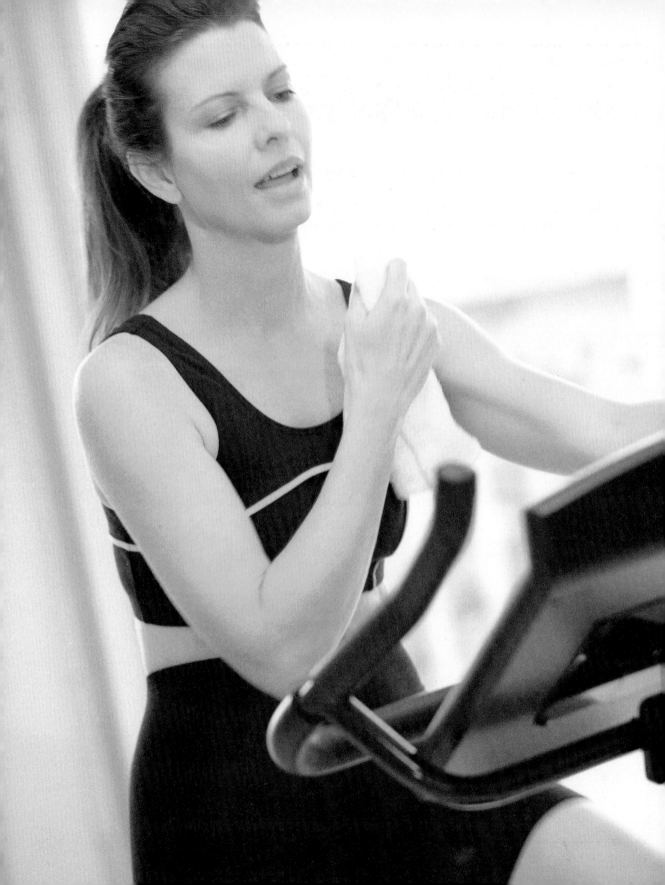

Chapter 5

Creating a Home Gym

CAN'T FIND A PLACE TO WORK OUT? How about exercising in the privacy of your own home? Creating a home gym can be as simple as stashing a couple of hand weights in your wardrobe or as complex as having an entire room full of equipment. Find out how to turn your home into a workout heaven without having to move all the furniture by using resistance bands, straps, and mats that can easily be packed up and hidden. No matter what your budget or space constrictions, there are many ways to exercise at home.

In this chapter...

✔ Make it easy to exercise any time

✔ Simple space savers

✔ Fun fitness videos

✔ A rundown on home cardio machines

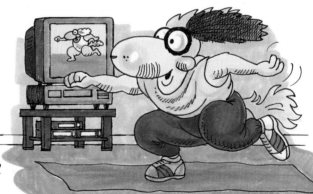

EXERCISING AT HOME IS A CONVENIENT AND TIME-SAVING ALTERNATIVE TO THE GYM

Make it easy to exercise any time

DON'T LIKE THE IDEA OF EXERCISING in a crowded gym? Don't have a street to run on, a bike or a pool nearby? That's no reason not to get or stay in shape! There's no excuse for not exercising when it's simple to create a home gym.

For beginners and experienced exercisers alike, working out at home is a convenient and time-saving alternative to the gym. You can avoid crowds, for one thing. If you work or live in a busy area, maybe the last thing you want to do is deal with more people. It's nice to have quiet time working out at home where you don't have to wait for machines – especially if you can go only during rush hour.

Exercising at home can give beginners or people who haven't recently worked out a head start on fitness so that they don't start out "cold" when they hit the gym. Some people are intimidated or feel self-conscious walking into a gym when they haven't worked out for a while. In your home gym, you can get re-acquainted with exercise and gain a little confidence before going public.

Having a choice

Even athletes benefit from the home gym. I know a professional cross-country skier who lifts weights or rides a stationary bike whenever she's at home watching television. By exercising while watching, she never feels guilty in front of the tube.

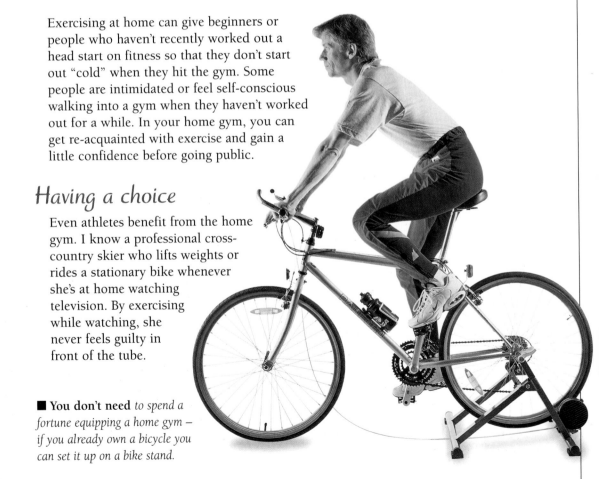

■ **You don't need** *to spend a fortune equipping a home gym – if you already own a bicycle you can set it up on a bike stand.*

The home gym is a great alternative if you can't get to the gym because you live too far away, or if you don't have the cash for a membership. And you can forget about the weather. Through rain, sleet, or snow, you can always work out at home. Even if you do have a gym membership, it's great to have an alternative if you can't go on a regular basis.

The most important thing is that you work out where you feel most comfortable.

Another benefit of exercising at home is that you can squeeze in a quick exercise session when you only have a few minutes. Some exercise is better than none.

One quick way to get a mini-workout is to set a kitchen timer for 20 minutes (or however long you have), put on your favourite record, and dance, stretch, or do push-ups – anything you like. Just keep moving until the buzzer rings.

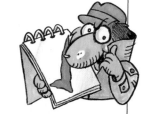

Simple space savers

CREATING A HOME GYM DOES *not mean you absolutely must go out and buy big pieces of exercise equipment. Whether you have a small flat where you have to move the furniture just to sneeze or whether you have an entire floor dedicated to fitness, there is a home workout strategy for everyone. Here is a list of some space-saving fitness items that are great if you don't have a lot of space, money, or time to set up a complete home gym. Later on in the book, we'll talk more about how you can incorporate these items into your workout.*

Resistance bands

A resistance band is the ultimate space-saving exercise item. Some resistance bands look like giant rubber bands, and some are rubber tubes with handles. They come in various lengths – the average length being about 1.5 metres (5 ft) long, – and in different resistance levels. These are good substitutes for or supplements to weights because they build muscle strength and provide all-over body toning.

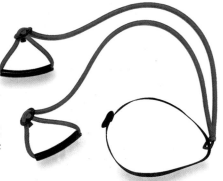

RESISTANCE BANDS

You can roll up a resistance band and throw it in a drawer when you're not using it. The bands are great for people who live in small flats or studios or who want to work out anywhere. They're cheap and extremely portable. For a few simple resistance band exercises, see Chapter 17.

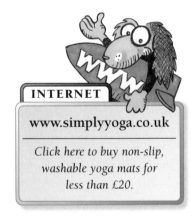

Straps

Straps are a great stretching aid because they allow you to extend your reach. They're similar to resistance bands, but there's no give. They're used everywhere from yoga classes to professional football training. (Next time you watch a game, watch the team stretching beforehand. You're likely to see straps being used.) Straps extend your reach and help you hold stretches for longer. They're especially good for hamstring, shoulder, and hip stretches.

Yoga mats

Yoga mats can be used for more than just yoga. They're great for stretching, especially if you don't feel like sweeping and mopping every time you want to flop down on the floor. Yoga mats provide a bit of cushioning to make those crunches a little more tolerable. Also, yoga mats are sticky, so they won't slip around as you're trying to touch your toes. Because you can roll them up easily, yoga mats are simple to carry and store.

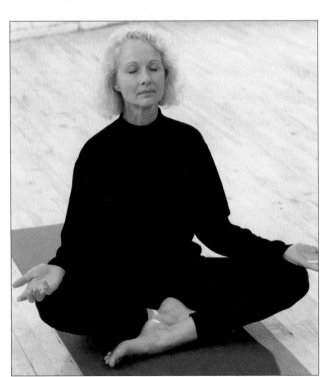

■ **Yoga mats** *are usually made from a piece of thin, rubberized material that fits the length of your body. Because they are sticky, they help you keep your hands and feet in position when doing exercises.*

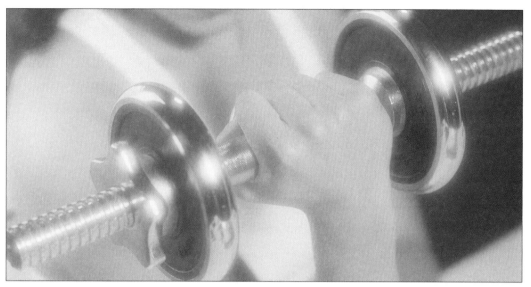

■ **Hand weights** *are extremely versatile. They come in different sizes and can be used at home or in the gym as part of your overall body conditioning routine.*

Hand weights

Hand weights, or *dumbbells*, don't take up much space, and yet they sculpt your arms and upper body. They can work your legs too, if you hold them while lunging, walking, or doing squats.

Women beginners should start off with 1.3–2.2 kg (3–5lb) weights, and beginning men should start with 3.6–6.8 kg (8–15lb) weights.

DEFINITION

Dumbbells *aren't what you call airheads; they are free weights designed to be held in one hand. They're usually used in pairs.*

Chin-up bar

This age-old contraption can really build upper-body strength. It is an overhead horizontal bar that can easily be installed in a doorway. You pull yourself up until your chin tops the bar. This action really builds muscle groups in the arms and back and is a good exercise for men; it's a bit more challenging for women. Some gyms have chin-up machines that help lift your body up so that the bar provides a challenge without being impossible. A chin-up bar may not be for you, so do try one out at the gym or at someone else's house before you buy.

INTERNET

www.bodyactive-
superstore.co.uk

Buy a chin-up bar for £14.99.

CHIN-UP BAR

Fun fitness videos

FITNESS VIDEOS CAN BE A HOOT. *They can teach you how to salsa dance, hula dance, weight-train, and many other offbeat ways to get some exercise. Like classes, they offer something for everyone. They cater to people at all levels from absolute beginners to advanced fitness junkies.*

Why use them?

I often hear people who've lost a lot of weight say they started at home with videos. Yes, you do need a small area on the floor, but still, one great thing about videos is that they're small and you can tuck them out of sight when you're not using them. Yet they're worth their weight in gold. I love learning new moves to add to my home workout through videos. Also, I find that trying to follow a fun video workout takes my mind away from the fact that I'm working out, and I just have fun. (Either that or I'm so busy trying to follow the steps that I'm not thinking about the sweat!)

If you have trouble following the steps and get confused trying to sync up left to right with the people on the screen, watch your fitness video in a mirror so as to be stepping with the same foot as the class.

Another reason to check the mirror while exercising with a video is that there's no one there to observe your form when you are learning a discipline (like dance or kickboxing for example) at home alone. So, watch yourself, if you can, to make sure you're doing the right moves correctly.

If you're taking a class, a video can be a helpful addition for days you can't make it. A video also offers you a chance to try something at home before going to a class.

What to look for

Most videos are targeted and labelled for beginning, intermediate, or advanced exercisers. In addition, most include modified versions of the workout, either more challenging or easier workouts, alongside the normal one. Some videos feature simple moves like push-ups and jumping jacks, while others involve complicated, highly choreographed dance

Trivia...

Actress Jane Fonda was one of the first to make exercise videos popular. Starting with Jane Fonda's Workout, she released many top-selling workout videos in the '80s and '90s.

INTERNET

www.amazon.co.uk

Click on "videos" or "DVDs" and then on the exercise and fitness, or family health and lifestyle sections to find out what's on offer in terms of home workouts.

moves. When I try a new dance workout video, I'm always secretly hoping that I'll learn some fun moves I can use on the dance floor. Usually that would only work if I were willing to drop and do 10 push-ups at the club! John Travolta would never approve.

Don't overdo it just because there's no one there to check on you. You should always monitor yourself and work at a pace that's comfortable for you no matter how hard the video works you.

What you need

For this you need a VCR and a small spot on the floor in front of the TV set. Make sure you have everything the video requires. Some require hand weights, a *stability ball*, a chair, or other specialized equipment.

> **DEFINITION**
>
> *A **stability ball**, also called a fitness ball or a Swiss ball, is a large rubber ball that is used to develop strength, flexibility, and balance.*

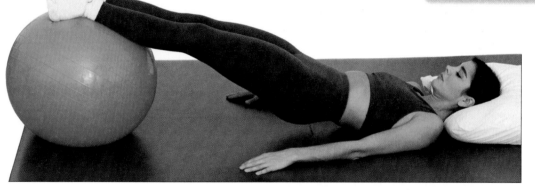

STABILITY BALL EXERCISE

With a little ingenuity, you can make some quick substitutions for items you don't have to hand: for example, if you don't have hand weights and you need them for a video, try holding 400g (16 oz) or heavier cans of food. It's not ideal, but it gets the job done. Also, if you don't have a mat, use a large towel.

Not every video suits everyone's needs. In your search for your own perfect video, it's a good idea to borrow from a friend or from the library before buying.

A good resource for fitness videos is Amazon's web site. Here you'll find a brief description of each video, plus reviews posted by people who've tried them out.

FITNESS VIDEOS

Reputable fitness videos are made by Karen Voight, Kathy Smith, and Denise Austin, to name a few. There are plenty more, so look around to find what's best for you. Here are a few ideas to get you started:

1 *Billy Blanks' Tae-Bo 1: The Future of Fitness*
World martial arts champ Billy Blanks instructs you in his own brand of fitness, Tae-Bo. This is basically martial arts and boxing moves (such as punching and kicking) turned into an aerobic dance-style workout. There's no equipment needed: just adequate space and bags of energy. It's quite strenuous but rewarding once you master the moves

2 *Keli Roberts – Total Body Circuit Training*
Keli Roberts presents her own personal total body circuit workout using step and resistance bands. The instructions are easy to follow and there are options along the way for beginners, so if you haven't used resistance bands before, this is a good way to learn. There's plenty to challenge more experienced exercisers, too, – if you can make it all the way through, you'll really feel like you've worked that body

3 *The Bootcamp Workout*
Phew! This new exercise regime, which is catching on in the UK after sweeping America, has military instructors putting you through rigorous army-style physical training. If you can cope with being shouted at and blasting through squat thrusts and star jumps (no slacking!), this might just be for you. But be warned: this is not for the fainthearted

4 *Barbara Currie's Yoga*
There are three routines on this video, with postures for beginners as well as more advanced positions. The first routine is an all-over body stretch that takes only 10 minutes. This is perfect if you're trying to fit in some exercise before going to work in the mornings

5 *Belly Dancing – a Fitness Programme*
A lesson in belly dancing!! This one is great for beginners because it's not physically challenging. It's a relaxing lesson with easy-to-follow moves that build up into a complete routine. Jacqueline Chapman is the instructor teaching you the basics, which once learned can be choreographed into your own routine. The sound quality isn't great, but don't let that put you off

A rundown on home cardio machines

IF YOU HAVE THE MONEY, TIME, and especially the space, a cardio machine can really make your home gym. Many of the cardio machines (we talked about them in Chapter 3) that you find in gyms can be purchased for home use. Although equipment for commercial use is more expensive, larger, and sturdier because it must stand up to multiple users, the machines you can buy for your home are similar in that they perform the same functions. Elliptical crosstrainers, treadmills, stationary bikes, stair climbers, and rowing machines can all be purchased for home use.

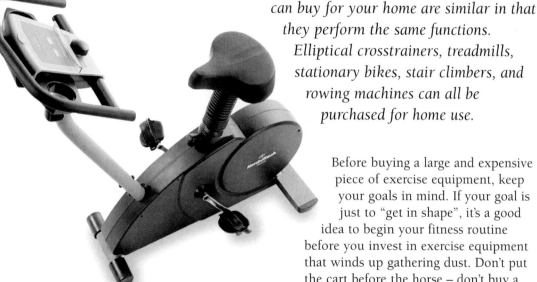

■ **A stationary bike** *is an expensive item of equipment, so be certain you'll use it before buying.*

Before buying a large and expensive piece of exercise equipment, keep your goals in mind. If your goal is just to "get in shape", it's a good idea to begin your fitness routine before you invest in exercise equipment that winds up gathering dust. Don't put the cart before the horse – don't buy a treadmill before you start running. You may find that swimming or even running outside is a better choice.

Features

You can find cheap exercise equipment, but do be aware that there is a correlation between price and quality. Some machines that cost less are cheap and flimsy. Then again, some machines with extra features that you may not need cost more, too. Most cardio machines will have speed, distance, and time-expended measurements on the console. That's all you really need, but some offer calories expenditure or built-in heart-rate monitors as well. People who are counting calories, or who want to make sure that they stay in their training zone, may want to spend more for these extras.

Try it before you buy it

If you can, join a gym even for a short period of time so you can experiment with various machines to see what style and features you like best. Ask around – if you have any friends who have home equipment, ask them whether they are happy with what they bought and if you can come over and try it. Once you've narrowed down your search, go to a shop that specializes in home exercise equipment. It's always best to try before you buy, so step on and get a feel for the machine you want to purchase.

Wear your workout clothes and athletic shoes to the shop so that you can give your prospects a test ride.

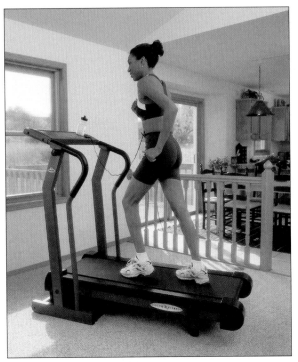

■ **Consider where** *you'll put your exercise equipment – check that you've got room for it before you buy.*

Before you go

Think about where your piece of exercise equipment will fit in your house or flat. Even small machines are going to need a little room to operate. Before you pick a spot, remember that you want to make it somewhere inviting.

A sunny living room is more inviting than a dank basement, but you have to make the best of what you have. If the only place you have is in the basement, then make it cosy by decorating, or by putting up soothing lighting.

Once you've found the place for your equipment, measure the vertical space as well as the floor space. Bring the measuring tape to the shop with you so you can be sure that what you choose will fit in your place.

Don't believe the hype

Be wary of equipment that promises too much. No one machine can do everything. Even if you have a cardio machine in your apartment, you're still going to need to strength train and stretch. Also, make sure the movement of the machine isn't a movement you could do without the machine. Many ab rollers, or other abdominal machines, don't offer anything you couldn't do with crunches or sit-ups.

There are many useless gadgets out there (as well as a lot of useful ones). I've been stuck with large pieces of equipment that I never used because I found I could do the same movement without them.

Also consider . . .

Another way to narrow down your search is by taking a careful look at the warranty. Make sure you know what repairs and maintenance are covered and for how long.

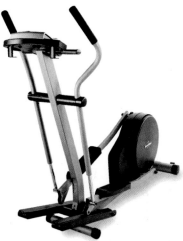

Check to see if there's any kind of trial period so you can be sure you're getting what you want.

Also, while taking a practice run, check: is the machine loud? Is it easy to operate? Does it offer a smooth ride? One element not to be underestimated is the aesthetic. Do you like the way it looks? This piece of equipment is going to be in your living space, so either it's got to look okay to you, or you should be able to hide it when it's not in use. Bear in mind that some machines are foldable. Make sure it's easy to fold or move if that's the way you're going to go.

■ **Make sure you like the look** *of an exercise machine if you're going to keep it in your living area.*

A simple summary

✔ Setting up a space to work out at home makes working out easy.

✔ A few simple items can help you get a workout without taking up a lot of space.

✔ Fitness videos can be a fun addition to anyone's routine.

✔ There are many things to consider before buying a cardio machine, such as a treadmill or stationary bike, for your home.

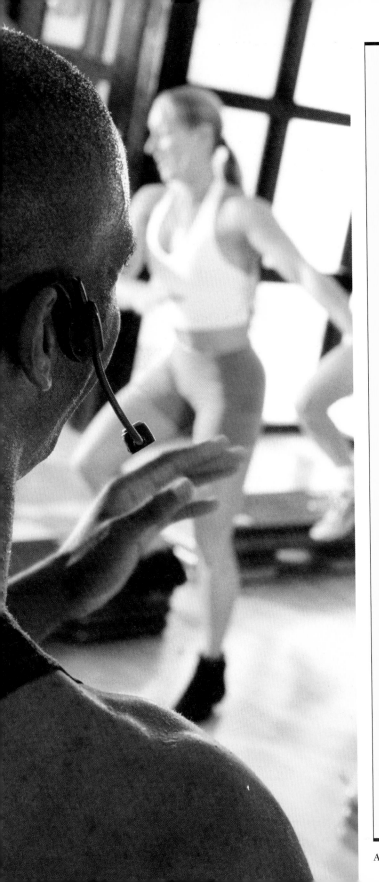

PART TWO

A WELL-ROUNDED ROUTINE IS KEY TO FITNESS

GETTING FIT

So HOW DO WE GO ABOUT getting in shape safely and intelligently? In this part, we'll break the workout down into simple and easy-to-understand (and do) sections. Find out why every exercise session should always include a *warm-up, stretch, and cool-down*. We'll 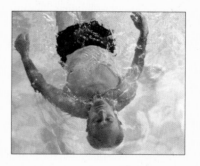 also talk about the kinds of exercise that combine to create a well-rounded fitness routine – *aerobic* exercise, *stretching*, and *strength training*.

Each chapter includes detailed descriptions and tips for beginners as well as a few workouts to try. Learn how to train to run a road race, do tai chi, and lift weights, to name just a few. This section will broaden your knowledge base in the universe of exercise and fitness so as to get you well on your way to being fit, healthy, and happy.

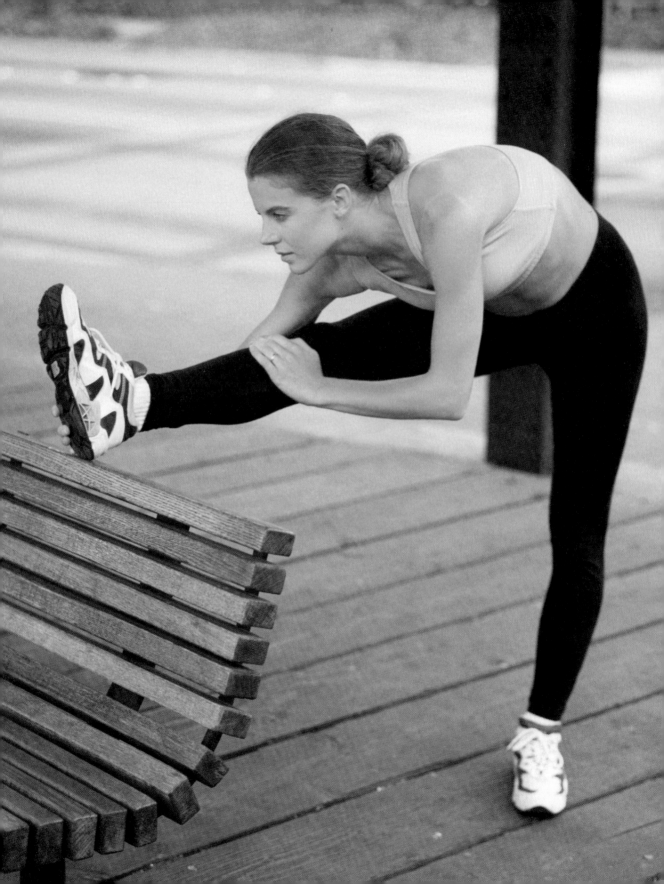

Chapter 6

Basic Elements of a Workout

EVERY EXERCISE SESSION should consist of four elements: warm up, stretch, work out, and cool down. In the actual session, these should be done all together and in order. For the purposes of this chapter, I'm going to break the session down and take a look at each element individually. At the end, we'll put it all together for a few simple workouts for the gym and home.

In this chapter...

✓ Warm it up

✓ Stretch it out

✓ Work it out

✓ Cool it down

✓ Put it all together

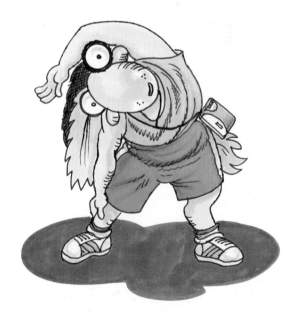

STRETCHING SHOULD FEATURE AT THE BEGINNING AND END OF EVERY EXERCISE SESSION

Warm it up

WARMING UP MEANS, *literally, raising your body temperature and warming up your muscles. It's important to warm up before stretching or exercising because working cold muscles can cause injuries. Imagine a rubber band. If you take a rubber band out of the freezer and immediately try to stretch it, it will probably snap in half as soon as you stretch it out a little. Now, take another rubber band and warm it up a little on a sunny windowsill; you'll probably have better luck stretching it out and snapping it back into place. Your muscles are like that rubber band; they need to be warmed up before use.*

Warming up with a few minutes of light exercise gradually increases the blood flow to the exercising muscles and reduces your chances of getting injured with strains, pulls, or other painful injuries. With a warm-up, muscles become more pliable and less likely to tear. I've noticed that if I go directly from sitting at the computer to skipping with cold muscles, my ankles hurt and feel weak; but if I warm them up a bit just by walking around first, they don't bother me in the least.

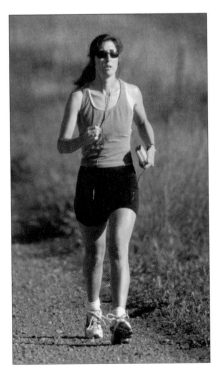

Starting slowly

You can, of course, take a warm bath or use a heating pad to warm up your muscles. That is better than nothing. But slowly going through the motions of the exercise you're about to do increases the blood flow to those specific areas and better prepares them for more rigorous exercise. If you're going to run, for example, warm up with a light 5- to 10-minute jog. Blood flow needs to increase substantially to protect the muscles from injury during exercise.

Working isolated muscle groups — such as doing push-ups — is not enough to get your whole body warmed up properly.

■ **About 5 to 10 minutes** *of brisk walking will help prepare your muscles for more intense exercise and protect them from injury when you're working out hard.*

All you need to do to warm up is move around slowly and easily for 5 or 10 minutes. Here are some simple ways to warm up:

- Brisk walk – for 5 minutes
- Light jog on road or treadmill
- Cycling – ride for 5 to 10 minutes in an easy gear on flat terrain
- Swimming – swim leisurely for 5 to 10 minutes
- Golf – 5 to 10 minutes of walking or putting
- Running – 5 to 10 minutes of easy jogging
- Leisurely walk – for 10 minutes
- Tennis – 5 to 10 minutes easy rally before match
- Roller skating – 5 to 10 minutes easy skating on flat terrain
- Dance for a few minutes

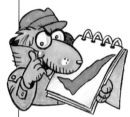

About 5 or 10 minutes of dancing wildly to your favourite song (by yourself if you need to) is a great all-over body warm-up because it not only raises your body temperature, it puts you in the right frame of mind for working out. It helps relax you and remind you that exercise isn't a chore – it's a lot of fun.

Stretch it out

ONCE YOUR MUSCLES ARE sufficiently warm, you are ready to stretch. In a nutshell, stretching is exercise that increases the range of motion for a muscle or joint. Although often neglected, stretching plays a vital role in overall fitness and health.

If you want to be sure for yourself that stretching after a little exercise is best, try stretching before and after you warm up. (Not too hard, though, please.) Which was easier? How far could you stretch warm muscles versus cold ones? Once again, think about that rubber band; a warm rubber band is much easier to stretch than a cold one.

Stretching is just as important as any other element of your exercise routine. Without stretching, you're more likely to strain and pull muscles and put extra wear and tear on joints. Stretching can also help prevent some post-workout soreness because strong, flexible, stretched muscles recover better than strong but stiff, unstretched muscles. Stretching also reduces muscle tension, and that in itself can make your whole body feel more relaxed.

Six simple stretches

These six stretches hit all the major muscle groups and are a good way to stretch before a workout – or any time. Repeat each stretch two or three times. For more stretches, check out *Stretching*, by Bob Anderson (Shelter Publications, 2000). This book is the ultimate guide to stretching, the one that fitness leaders and doctors often recommend. It includes stretches for daily activities as well as stretches for particular sports.

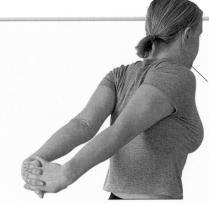

Remember to keep your chin in and your chest out

1 Chest

From a standing position, interlace your fingers behind your back. Slowly turn elbows inwards while straightening your arms, stretching your shoulders, arms, and chest. Hold for 5 to 10 seconds. If that's fairly easy, lift your arms up behind you until you feel the stretch in your arms, shoulders, and chest. Hold for 5 to 10 seconds.

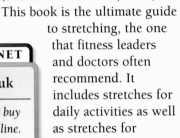

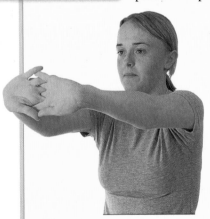

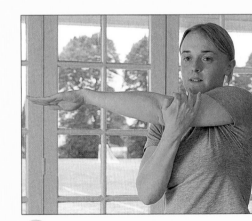

2 Back

From a standing position, interlace your fingers out in front of you at shoulder height. Turn palms outwards and extend your arms, pushing out with your hands. You should feel the stretch in your shoulders, middle of your upper back, arms, hands, fingers, and wrists. Hold for 15 seconds. Relax and repeat.

3 Shoulder

Standing or sitting, stretch your shoulder and the middle of your upper back by gently pulling your left elbow across your chest towards the right shoulder. Keep your shoulders level with each other and down (not tense and up by your ears). You should feel the stretch in your left shoulder. Hold for 10 seconds and repeat with your right arm.

4 Calf

Standing a few feet away from a wall, lean on it with your forearms, head resting on your hands. Step with your right leg towards the wall, bending your right knee, and keep your left leg straight behind. Move your hips forwards, keeping your lower back flat and the heel of your left leg on the ground, toes pointed straight ahead. You should feel the stretch in your left calf. Hold for 10 to 15 seconds, change legs and repeat. To go further into the stretch, bend your right leg more.

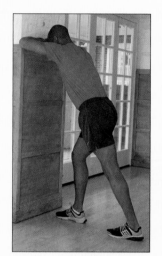

5 Quadriceps

To stretch your **quadriceps**, bring your left foot behind you and, holding the top of your left foot with your left hand, pull towards your buttocks. Stand straight, tilting hips slightly forwards. Put your right hand on a wall or support, and as your balance improves, hold your right arm straight out to the side. You should feel this stretch in your left thigh. Hold for 10 to 20 seconds, change legs, and repeat.

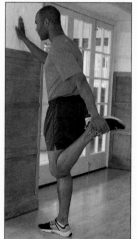

> **DEFINITION**
>
> The **quadriceps** are the muscles in the front of the thigh. The term is often shortened to "quads".
> The **hamstring** is the group of muscles and tendons that runs behind your knee and thigh.

6 Hamstring

To stretch your **hamstring**, lie flat on your back, and raise your right leg straight above you at 90 degrees, keeping your left leg flat on the floor. (If it's more comfortable or if you have lower back trouble, bend your left knee and put your left foot on the floor.) Keep your lower back flat against the floor. Hold your right leg with your hands right behind the knee for support. Pull slightly with your hands towards your head to feel a stretch along the back of your thigh. Hold for 30 seconds. Switch sides.

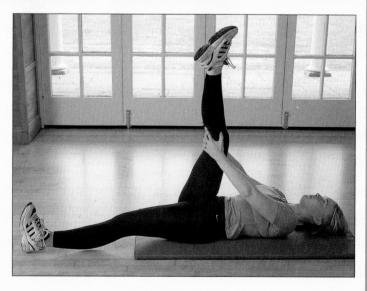

Tips for stretching

When you stretch, make sure you stretch your entire body, focusing on areas that you're about to exercise most vigorously. Swimmers should give the shoulders extra attention while runners need to focus on stretching their legs thoroughly. For a general, overall workout, proper stretching means stretching all the major muscle groups including your back, chest, legs, and shoulders. Stretching should feel good; it should never hurt. You may feel tension, but pain – especially a sharp pain – while stretching means you're extending too far and could be doing more harm than good.

Don't bounce! Jerky, bouncy movements actually tighten the muscles you're trying to stretch.

In general, hold each stretch for about 20 seconds to let the muscles fully relax. For the first 10 seconds, stretch mildly, getting comfortable in the position. For the next 10 seconds, move slowly deeper into the stretch as you breathe deeply. The tension should subside. If it doesn't, ease off a little. If the tension becomes more intense or feels painful as you hold it, you're stretching too far. Some of the stretches on the previous pages don't need to be held for the entire 20 seconds, but you can increase the amount of time as you progress.

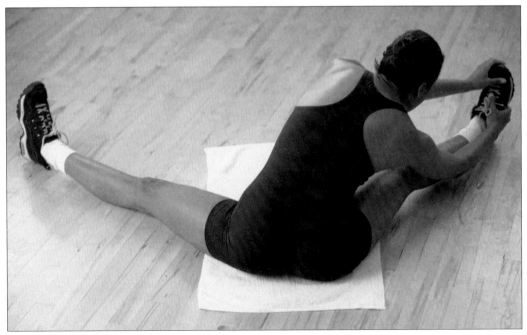

■ **If you're about to go running,** *focus on stretching your leg muscles after an initial warm-up. With regular stretching, you'll protect yourself against pulled muscles and strained joints.*

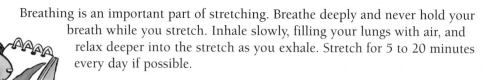

Breathing is an important part of stretching. Breathe deeply and never hold your breath while you stretch. Inhale slowly, filling your lungs with air, and relax deeper into the stretch as you exhale. Stretch for 5 to 20 minutes every day if possible.

The key to successful stretching is regularity and relaxation.

Work it out

ANY EXERCISE ROUTINE *should include a combination of stretching, aerobic conditioning, and* **strength training**. *Sometimes a nice long stretching session might be your exercise for the day. Yoga, for example, is an excellent way to get a great stretch. A session of yoga can provide enough exercise for one day. We'll talk about yoga and other disciplines in Chapter 9.*

DEFINITION

Strength training *refers to weight-bearing or resistance exercise. For more about strength training, see Chapter 10.*

Whether the workouts you are doing are aerobic or strength training, you need to warm up and stretch before starting. Any time you're going to exercise, whether it's a workout at the gym or playing a sport, it's important to include every element – the warm-up, stretch, and cool-down – as part of your exercise session. It's the fastest and safest way to get fit. Although it might be tempting to go on a run or play a game of football without warming up or stretching, you're putting yourself at a higher risk of injury when you do that. A well-rounded exercise routine is worth the extra time spent.

■ **The fluid, unhurried movements** *of yoga enable you to practise beneficial stretching. Classic yoga postures like the one shown here (a variation of the Triangle pose) improve muscle tone and flexibility.*

Cool it down

COOLING DOWN AT THE END *of a workout means slowing down and gradually lowering your heart rate. It's not a good idea to stop suddenly because you could become faint or light-headed. Cooling down is very similar to warming up; in fact many of the same rules apply. The big difference is that it comes post- instead of pre-workout.*

The easiest way to cool down is by continuing the activity you've been doing – but at a much slower pace – before stopping. This cool-down can help prevent after-workout stiffness and soreness. Most cardio machines have an automatic warm-up and cool-down feature. I like to think of the cool-down as the dessert. If you want to think in food terms, the warm-up is the soup, the stretch is the appetizer, the workout is the main meal, and the cool-down is dessert.

After cooling down, stretch again. Even if you stretched very thoroughly before the workout, it's good to stretch again once your muscles are totally warmed up. You'll probably find you can go much further into the stretches after working out. Treat your body with at least a quick post-workout stretch before you hit the showers.

Put it all together

USING WHAT WE'VE LEARNED *about gyms, working out at home, and using these four elements of an exercise session, read on to find eight simple beginner workouts to try. These should help you get a feel for how to incorporate warming up, stretching, working out, and cooling down into every exercise session.*

Play it safe

You should consult your doctor before embarking on any fitness regimen, especially if any of the following describes you:

- You are a man over 45
- You are a woman over 55

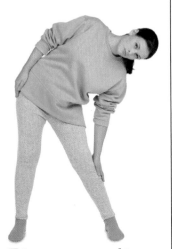

■ **Incorporate stretching** *into every exercise session, be it at home, at the gym, or outdoors.*

- You have a family history of heart disease or stroke
- You have diabetes
- You have high blood pressure
- You have high cholesterol
- You've recently had surgery
- You're pregnant
- You've led a mostly sedentary life

For tips on exercise for people with special needs and situations, see Chapter 16.

When you begin to exercise, pay close attention to your body. The safest way to start an exercise programme is at a low intensity and only until your legs or arms ache or feel heavy. If your muscles ache after a few minutes, then the first workouts should last only that long. As you get in better shape, you'll be able to work out for longer periods.

Simple beginner workouts

Here's my selection of straightforward beginner workouts to get you into the swing of warming up, stretching, working out, cooling down, and stretching again.

GYM WORKOUT 1

Warm-up: Walk briskly to the gym. (If it's really cold outside, you may need to do an additional warm up in the gym.)
Stretch: Find a mat and go through the six stretches (see pages 102–103).
Workout: Jog lightly on treadmill (no incline) for 15 minutes.
Cool-down: Walk briskly on treadmill for 5 minutes.
Stretch: Quick stretch, concentrating on legs.

GYM WORKOUT 2

Warm-up: Lightly jog around track, 5 to 10 minutes.
Stretch: Do the six stretches.
Workout: Work at moderate pace on elliptical cross trainer for 15 minutes.
Cool-down: Go slowly on the cross trainer for 5 minutes.
Stretch: 5 minutes, making sure you stretch quads.

GYM WORKOUT 3

Warm-up:	Walk in place and move your arms back and forth across your upper body for a few minutes.
Stretch:	Do the six stretches.
Workout:	Work at moderate pace on rowing machine for 15 minutes.
Cool-down:	Row slowly for 5 minutes.
Stretch:	5 minutes, concentrating on arms.

GYM WORKOUT 4

Warm-up:	Ride lightly on stationary bike (no resistance) for 5 to 10 minutes.
Stretch:	10 minutes.
Workout:	Ride at moderate speed for 15 minutes.
Cool-down:	Ride slowly for 5 minutes.
Stretch:	5 minutes.

GYM WORKOUT 5

Warm-up:	Jog or walk briskly on treadmill for 5 to 10 minutes.
Stretch:	Do the six stretches.
Workout:	Work at moderate pace on stair climber for 15 minutes.
Cool-down:	Go slowly on stair climber for 5 minutes.
Stretch:	Concentrate on legs.

Most fitness classes include a warm-up, stretch, workout, and cool-down. If you're going to be late, or if it's your first time to a class, warm up and stretch before going in or take time in the room to warm up and stretch before joining in.

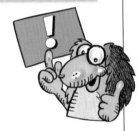

POOL WORKOUT

Warm-up:	Swim slow laps for 5 to 10 minutes.
Stretch:	In the water, stretch arms, legs, and back.
Workout:	Swim laps at a moderate pace for 15 minutes.
Cool-down:	Swim slow laps for 5 minutes.
Stretch:	Out of the water, stretch for 10 minutes.

HOME WORKOUT

Home is a great place to take your time with stretching, especially if it's peaceful and no one is around. Be decadent with your stretching when you're at home.

Warm-up: Jog in place for 5 to 10 minutes.

Stretch: 15 minutes. Put a mat or towel on the floor for floor stretches.

Workout: Dance to five songs.

Cool-down: Walk in place or dance slowly.

Stretch: Stretch slowly and breathe deeply. Make sure you stretch your calves.

VIDEO WORKOUT

Most exercise videos include a warm-up on the tape. To be on the safe side, you might warm up and stretch a little before starting.

Warm-up: Jog in place for a few minutes.

Stretch: 5 minutes.

Workout: Participate in the exercise video.

Cool-down: Good tapes include a cool-down. If yours doesn't, make sure you continue light activity for a few minutes.

Stretch: If you have time, include a long stretch session after the video.

A simple summary

✓ Warming up your body with a little light activity is the way to begin any exercise.

✓ Stretching is an often neglected, yet vital, aspect of any workout.

✓ Workouts consist of aerobic exercise or strength training.

✓ After working out, cool your body down by slowing to a gradual stop.

✓ Check out a few workouts that incorporate warming up, stretching, working out, and cooling down.

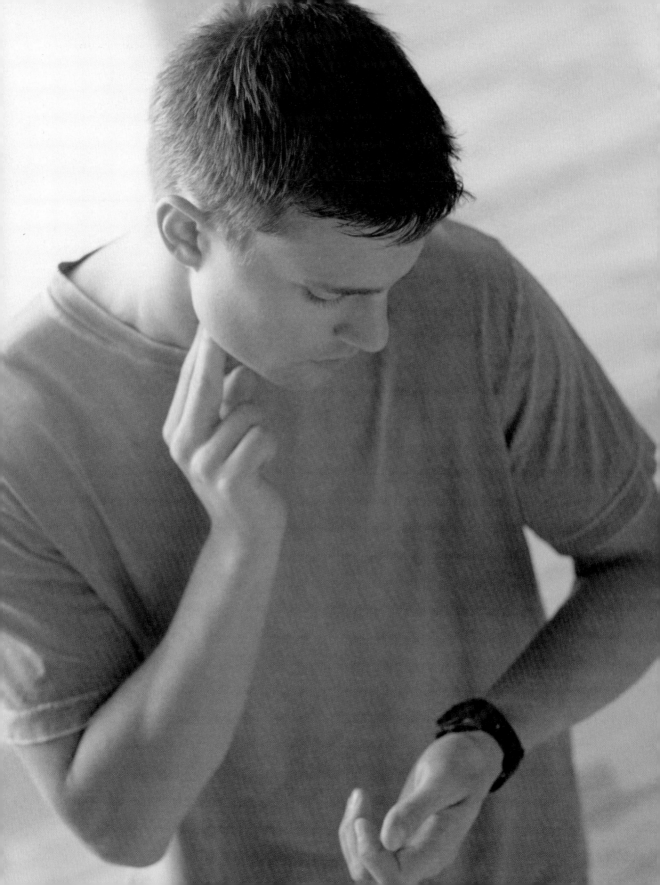

Chapter 7

Get Heart Smart

THE HEART, THE MOST VITAL ORGAN OF ALL, plays a major role in physical fitness. For one thing, aerobic exercise can greatly reduce your chances of getting heart disease. And monitoring your heart while you exercise is an excellent way to work out safely and effectively; it's a great measure of workout intensity. Read on to discover how to use your heart rate to help you gauge when you're exercising too hard or not hard enough for maximum benefits. Also, try the heart smart quiz at the end of the chapter to test what you know about heart health and physical fitness.

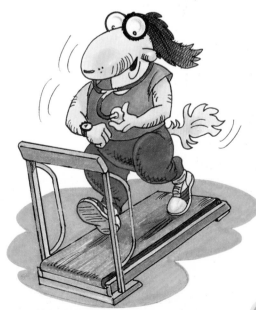

In this chapter...

✓ *The heart of the matter*

✓ *Measure your heart rate*

MEASURE YOUR HEART RATE AND ADJUST THE INTENSITY OF YOUR WORKOUT ACCORDINGLY

The heart of the matter

IT'S IMPOSSIBLE TO TALK about fitness and exercise without mentioning the heart and the cardiovascular system. As I mentioned in Chapter 1, aerobic exercise (exercise that gets your heart pumping and your blood moving) is one of the best ways to improve cardiovascular health. Since heart disease claims many lives each year, improving your heart health can help you lead a long, healthy life.

The heart itself is the "centre" of the cardiovascular system. It is a muscular, fist-sized organ that lies in the centre of your chest. Both the right and left sides have upper chambers (atria), which collect blood, and lower chambers (ventricles), which eject blood. The heart collects oxygen-depleted blood and pumps it into the lungs, where blood picks up oxygen and drops off carbon dioxide. The heart also pumps oxygen-rich blood to all the body's organs and cells.

HOW THE BLOOD GETS AROUND

Blood travels throughout the body via a complex system of blood vessels. Arteries carry blood away from the heart. They're small and strong and bear the highest blood pressure. Veins carry blood back to the heart. They're a little larger in diameter than arteries, and carry the same amount of blood but at a slower speed. Capillaries are hairlike vessels that distribute blood to outlying areas.

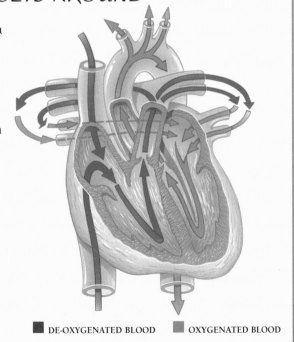

■ **Blood vessels** *connected to the heart carry blood to and from all body parts. De-oxygenated (oxygen-depleted) blood is pumped through the heart to the lungs. Oxygenated (oxygen-rich) blood is then pumped back to the heart and all around the body.*

■ DE-OXYGENATED BLOOD ■ OXYGENATED BLOOD

Since every bodily organ thrives on oxygen, maintaining a strong heart is crucial to overall health.

A note about blood pressure

Blood pressure is the force of blood against the walls of the arteries. Blood pressure in a normal range is great for heart health, while high blood pressure is definitely unhealthy.

High blood pressure makes the heart pump with more force, in turn forcing the arteries to carry blood that is moving under great pressure. If high blood pressure continues for a long time, the heart and arteries may not function well and other organs could be affected.

And, with high blood pressure, there's an increased risk of stroke, heart failure, kidney failure, and heart attack.

Most people with high blood pressure have no symptoms, so it is important to get your blood pressure checked periodically.

That's the bad news. So what's the good news? Exercise can help! Physical fitness reduces your chances of heart disease by lowering your blood pressure and by keeping your heart strong and healthy.

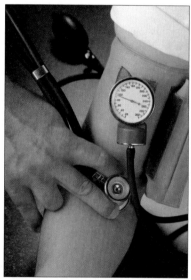

■ **Get early warning** *of any changes in your blood pressure by having regular checks with your doctor.*

HEART ATTACK SYMPTOMS

Although it's usually men who have heart attacks, plenty of women have them, too. The problem is that women don't always get to the doctor quickly enough because they don't realize they're having a heart attack.

While the classic symptoms of a heart attack include sharp chest pain, tightness or heaviness in the chest, and shortness of breath, many women have little to no chest pain and feel nausea and extreme fatigue while having a heart attack.

Why do we need aerobic exercise?

Aerobic exercise provides many of the benefits we talked about in Chapter 1. It makes you more resilient against sickness, disease, and fatigue, and also reduces tension and improves mood.

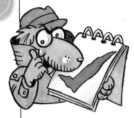

Aerobic exercise, in particular, builds endurance, improves cardiovascular health, and is the best and fastest way to lose weight.

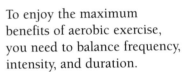

Trivia...

The heart pumps about 6 litres (10.5 pints) of blood around the body each minute. During exercise, not only is the blood pumped at a much faster rate, but as much as 12 times the normal volume of blood is routed to the muscles.

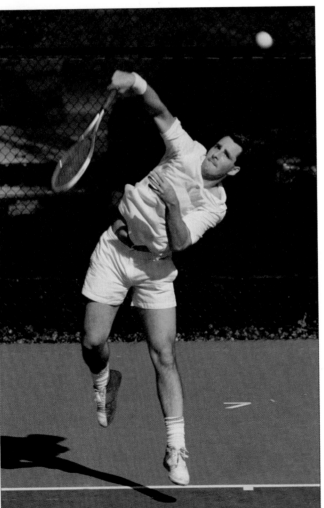

To enjoy the maximum benefits of aerobic exercise, you need to balance frequency, intensity, and duration.

Frequency and duration are rather easy to measure, because frequency refers to how often you exercise, and duration refers to how long you exercise. Intensity is best measured by how hard your heart is working.

■ **Tennis is a great aerobic** *exercise. If you play fairly regularly you'll develop a good level of aerobic fitness, which in turn will help guard against heart disease and stress-related illnesses.*

Measure your heart rate

THE BEST WAY TO MEASURE *your workout intensity is by monitoring your heart rate. Your heart rate is basically your pulse. Your target heart rate is what your heart rate should be while you are exercising. Staying within your target heart rate can help you have productive, safe workouts.*

If you're exercising too far below your target heart rate, you won't reap all the benefits of exercise. But if you're too far above it, you're going to get tired and overheated, and you're more likely to injure yourself. Beginners who exercise too hard, too fast are often the ones to drop out.

Heart-rate monitors, as mentioned in Chapter 4, provide a handy way to check your heart rate. But you can also measure your heart rate on your own.

Equation for a good workout

An easy way to identify your target heart rate is by figuring out your age-predicted maximum heart rate.

 Figure out your maximum heart rate: Subtract your age from 220. 220 – age = maximum heart rate in beats per minute.

220 is our maximum heart rate at birth.

If you're 30 years old, your maximum heart rate is 190 beats per minute (220 – 30 = 190).

 Find your target heart rate: A good target heart rate to aim for is 55–90 per cent of your maximum heart rate. To find that number, multiply your maximum heart rate by .55 for the low end of your target heart-rate zone. Multiply your maximum heart rate by .90 for the high end of your target heart-rate zone.

To determine the target heart rate for a 30-year-old, take the maximum heart rate, 190 (220 minus the person's age), and multiply that by .55, which equals 104.5. That's the low end. For the high end, multiply 190 by .90, which equals 171. The target heart-rate zone for a 30-year-old is 104 to 171 heartbeats per minute.

Heart-rate charts and zones

If maths isn't your best subject, don't worry. Most gyms post heart-rate zone charts (or you can use the one below). All you have to do is check your pulse rate and compare it to the chart. Most charts show the following zones:

a **Red-line zone:** the top of most heart-rate charts will show the red-line zone, which is 90–100 per cent of your maximum heart rate (MHR)

Stay out of the "red-line" zone, or 90–100 per cent of your maximum heart rate. That's too high for anybody.

b *Anaerobic-***threshold zone:** in the anaerobic zone, over 90 per cent of your maximum heart rate, you're working out so hard that your cardiovascular system can't get oxygen to the muscles. Working out at this level is for serious athletes in training and should be done only under supervision

> **DEFINITION**
>
> Anaerobic *means without oxygen.*

HEART-RATE ZONES

If you don't want to do the calculations, just look for your age range, decide which zone you want to train in, and aim to push your pulse up to that rate during exercise.

Age	50% MHR	60% MHR	70% MHR	80% MHR	90% MHR	100% MHR
18–25	99	119	139	159	179	199
26–30	95	115	134	153	172	192
31–36	93	112	130	149	168	187
37–42	90	108	126	144	162	180
43–50	86	103	121	138	155	173
51–58	83	99	116	133	149	166
59–65	79	95	110	126	142	159
65+	76	91	106	121	136	152

c **Aerobic zone:** to improve aerobic capacity or athletic performance, aim for an intensity of 70–80 per cent of your maximum heart rate. That means 133 to 152 beats per minute for a 30-year-old

d **Weight-management zone:** to lose weight, the intensity should be at 60–70 per cent of your maximum heart rate. For a 30-year-old, that would be at about 114 to 133 beats per minute

e **Heart-health zone:** this is 50–60 per cent of your maximum heart rate, and is a gentle way to give your heart a workout. Someone who is just starting out, and whose goals are to get in better shape, should start exercising at this pace. For a 30-year-old, that would be 95 to 114 beats per minute

Aim to work out in your target heart-rate zone for about 20 minutes.

Taking your pulse

To take your own pulse (to find your heart rate beats per minute), place two fingers on your neck just below the jaw line or on the inside of your wrist. Wherever you can best feel your pulse is fine. Count your heartbeat for 30 seconds, then double it to get the beats per minute.

Some people choose to gauge their workout intensity by how they feel or by their perceived level of exertion. This is an alternative for people who don't have any heart concerns. Beginners who are embarking upon a strenuous new exercise routine, people who want to lose weight, and people who have had or who are susceptible to heart disease should pay special attention to their heart rate.

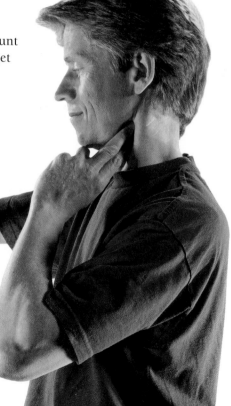

■ **Check your heart rate** *during exercise to make sure that it falls within the zone specified for your chosen level of activity.*

ARE YOU HEART SMART?

Test how much you know about how physical activity affects your heart. The following 12 statements are either true or false. Decide what you think, then compare your responses with the answers given below.

1 **Regular physical activity can reduce your chances of getting heart disease**

Heart disease is almost twice as likely to develop in inactive people, so this is true. Being physically inactive is a risk factor for heart disease along with cigarette smoking, high blood pressure, high blood cholesterol, and being overweight. The more risk factors you have, the greater your chance of getting heart disease. Regular physical activity (even mild to moderate exercise) can reduce this risk

2 **Most people get enough physical activity from their normal daily routines**

Since most people are very busy but not very active, this statement is false. Every adult should make a habit of getting 30 minutes of low to moderate levels of physical activity daily. This includes walking, gardening, and walking up stairs. If you are inactive now, begin by doing a few minutes of activity each day. If you engage in some activity only once in a while, try to work something into your routine every day. (For suggestions, check out "Moves that make a difference" in Chapter 1)

3 **You don't have to train like a marathon runner to become more physically fit**

This is true. Low- to moderate-intensity activities, such as pleasure walking, stair climbing, gardening, moderate to heavy housework, dancing, and home exercises can have both short- and long-term benefits. If you are inactive, the key is to get started. One great way is to take a walk for 10 to 15 minutes during your lunch break or take you dog for a walk every day

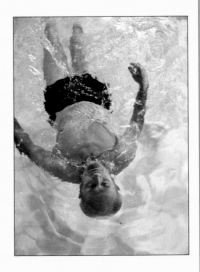

■ **Enjoy your exercise breaks.** *Regular swimming is a great way to keep your heart and lungs healthy.*

4   **Exercise programmes do not require a lot of time to be very effective**

It's true – it takes only a few minutes a day to become more physically active. If you don't have 30 minutes in your schedule for an exercise break, try to find two 15-minute periods or even three 10-minute periods. Once you discover how much you enjoy these exercise breaks, they'll become a habit you can't live without

At least 30 minutes of physical activity every day can help improve your heart health and lower your risk of heart disease.

5   **People who need to lose some weight are the only ones who will benefit from regular physical activity**

This statement is false. People who engage in regular physical activity experience many positive benefits. Regular physical activity gives you more energy, reduces stress, helps you to relax, and helps you to sleep better. It helps to lower high blood pressure and improves blood cholesterol levels. Physical activity helps to tone your muscles, burns off calories to help you lose extra pounds or stay at your desirable weight, and helps control your appetite. It can also increase muscle strength, help your heart and lungs work more efficiently, and let you enjoy your life more fully

6   **All exercises give you the same benefits**

False again. Low-intensity activities – if performed daily – can have some long-term health benefits and can lower your risk of heart disease. Regular, brisk, and sustained exercise for at least 30 minutes, 3 to 4 times a week, such as brisk walking, jogging, or swimming, is necessary to improve the efficiency of your heart and lungs and burn off extra calories. These kinds of activities are aerobic. Other activities may give you other benefits, such as increased flexibility or muscle strength, depending on the type of activity

7   **The older you are, the less active you need to be**

Although we tend to become less active with age, physical activity is still important, so this is false. In fact, regular physical activity in older people increases their capacity to continue everyday activities. In general, older people benefit from regular exercise just as young people do. What is important, no matter what your age, is tailoring the activity programme to your fitness level

8 **It doesn't take a lot of money or expensive equipment to become physically fit**

It's true – many activities require little or no equipment. For example, brisk walking requires only a comfortable pair of walking shoes. Also, many leisure centres have large pools, and a large number now offer inexpensive gym and weight training facilities and physical activity classes. Check with your local council to see what sports facilities and activities are available in your area

9 **There are many risks and injuries that can occur with exercise**

This is false. The most common risk in exercising is injury to the muscles and joints. Exercising too hard for too long usually causes such injuries, particularly if a person has been inactive for some time. To avoid injury, try to build up your level of activity gradually, listen to your body for early warning pains, be aware of possible signs of heart problems (such as pain or pressure in the left or mid-chest area, left neck, shoulder, or arm during or just after exercising, or sudden light-headedness, cold sweat, pallor, or fainting), and be prepared for special weather conditions

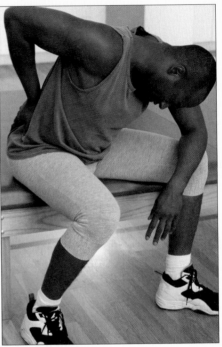

■ **Painful muscular injuries** *can be avoided by pacing yourself when exercising.*

10 **You should always consult a doctor before starting a physical activity programme**

This is true. You should ask your doctor before you start (or greatly increase) your physical activity if you: have a medical condition such as high blood pressure; have pains or pressure in the chest and shoulder area; tend to feel dizzy or faint; get very breathless after mild exertion; are middle-aged or older and have not been physically active or plan a fairly vigorous activity programme. If none of these apply, start slowly and get moving

11 **People who have had a heart attack should not start any physical activity programme**

Regular, physical activity can help reduce your risk of having another heart attack, so this is false. People who include regular physical activity in their lives after a heart attack improve their chances of survival and can improve how they feel and look. If you have had a heart attack, consult your doctor to be sure you are following a safe and effective exercise programme that will help prevent heart pain and further damage from overexertion

12 **To help you stay physically active, you should include a variety of activities**

This is true: pick several different activities that you like doing. You will be more likely to stay with your exercise plan if you enjoy the activities. Plan short-term as well as long-term goals. Keep a record of your progress, and check it regularly to see the progress you have made. Get your family and friends to join in. They can help keep you going

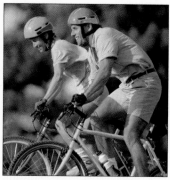

This quiz is adapted, with permission, from the US National Heart, Lung, and Blood Institute.

■ **Vary your routine** *and include activities you can share with friends and family.*

A simple summary

✔ Your heart is one of the most important parts of your body.

✔ Aerobic workouts are the best way to keep your heart healthy and happy.

✔ Exercising within your target heart-rate zone can make your workouts more productive.

✔ The heart health quiz is a test of your knowledge about heart health and physical activity. The answers confirm what you do know and fill in the gaps.

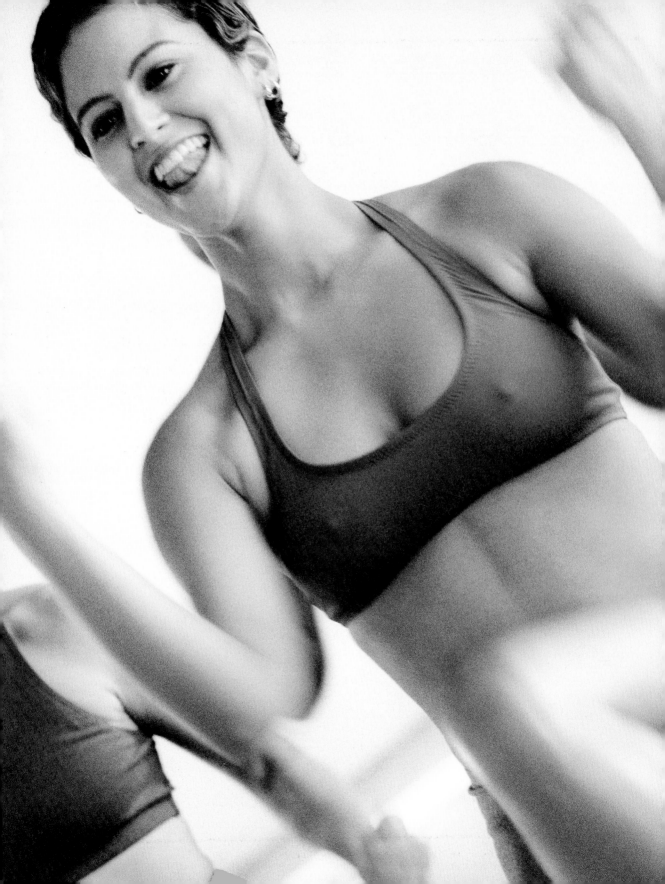

Chapter 8

Best Ways to Burn Calories

AEROBIC EXERCISE IS THE BEST WAY to burn calories and lose weight. Although aerobic dancing is certainly a fun way to exercise, there are plenty of other ways to get an aerobic workout. Any endurance exercise is aerobic and that includes running, cycling, swimming, and many team sports. The most important thing is that you find some aerobic activity you enjoy. Read on to find out which exercise suits you best and to pick up training tips on how to improve your performance.

In this chapter...

✔ Burning calories

✔ Walk before you run

✔ Running

✔ Cycling

✔ In the pool

✔ Team sports

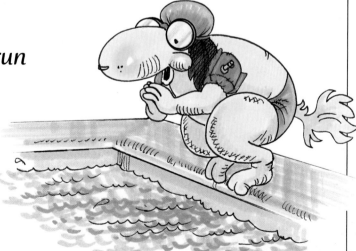

AEROBIC DANCING IS JUST ONE WAY TO BURN CALORIES AND SHED WEIGHT

Burning calories

THE EXACT NUMBER OF CALORIES you burn during exercise
is affected by your body weight, intensity of the workout, your level of
conditioning (how fit you are), and your metabolism. A person who is out of
shape and weighs more will burn more calories than a fit person who weighs
less. That's good news if you're trying to lose weight – the more you weigh,
the more calories you burn when you exercise. Also, the more effort you put
into your workout, the more calories you burn.

Keeping those variables in mind, here is a list of activities discussed in this chapter and
how many calories they burn per hour. These are calculated for a moderately fit person
who weighs 70 kilos (155 pounds), so if you weigh less than that, you'll burn fewer
calories and if you weigh more, you'll burn more. This is based on an hour of activity, so
if you walk for only half an hour, for example, cut the number of calories burned in half.

CALORIES BURNED DURING EXERCISE

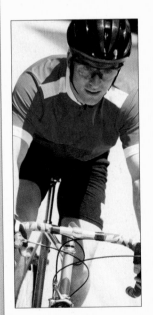

PEDAL POWER

Activity	Calories per hour*
Walking, moderate pace	246
Jogging, general	493
Running, general	563
Running, race speed	1267
Cycling, leisure	281
Cycling, race	1126
Mountain biking	598
Swimming laps, light to moderate effort	563
Water aerobics	281
Basketball	563
Football	493
Rugby	704
Ice hockey	563
Rounders or baseball	352
Volleyball	211
Golf	250

*(based on a 70 kg/155 lb person)

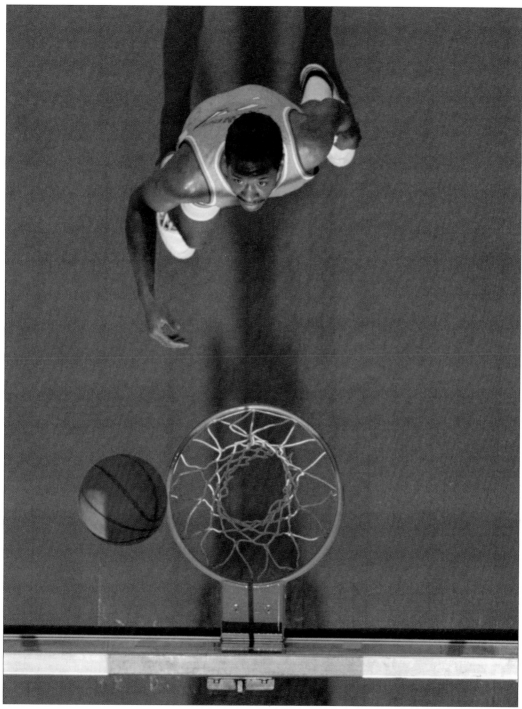

■ **Basketball is one sport** *that can help get you in shape. For a person who weighs 70 kilos (155 lbs), an hour spent running around the court will burn off around 560 calories.*

Walk before you run

IF YOU'RE JUST STARTING TO EXERCISE, *try walking first to ease into a routine. If you're overweight, or haven't exercised for a while, walking is an easy, non-impact way to get fit. Enlist a few friends and make it a social activity. This way you're having fun while being accountable to someone else, and you won't work out too hard because you'll need to be able to carry on a conversation as you stroll. (See "talk test" in Chapter 2.)*

Walking can be an end unto itself, or it can be a way to ease into jogging and running.

Running or walking a mile burns about 100 calories.

Walking very slowly won't make you super fit, but it's a great way to condition yourself to separate the time and mental space for exercise, and to prepare your body for running. (If that's what you want to do.) Start slowly. For the first week, start off by walking every other day (or whenever you can) for 15 minutes. Then you can begin to add frequency and duration. Try walking every day, and try walking for 20 then 30 minutes at a time.

Tips for walkers

- Keep your shoulders down and your back straight
- Bend both elbows to 90-degree angles
- Pump your arms front to back as you walk. (This may sound obvious, but I've seen people try to keep their arms still)
- Keep your stride at a natural length
- Point your toes straight ahead
- Don't lean forward

■ **Stepping out with friends** *is a good way to start a fitness campaign if you haven't exercised for some time. Go slowly at first and gradually speed up.*

Fitness walking, which basically means walking regularly at a good pace, is an excellent fitness routine. If you're ready for a new challenge, try running.

Since everybody is different, it might take weeks or months to get used to walking. Always go at your own pace and pay close attention to how you feel.

Once you feel comfortable with your walking routine, begin mixing in a little light jogging. If you've been walking 20 minutes a day for a week or two, and you're feeling pretty good, try running for 5 minutes and walking for 15. Gradually increase your running time, as you feel comfortable, until you're running for 15 minutes.

Gradual training is the key to long-term success.

Running

RUNNING OR JOGGING IS ONE *of the best and easiest ways to lose weight. It burns more calories than many other forms of exercise, and it's convenient – just throw on a pair of shoes and a comfy tracksuit and go!*

But running isn't for everyone. The high impact can be jarring and hard on joints. If you have chronic knee or lower back problems, you should stick to walking or another low-impact activity such as swimming.

Tips for runners

- As far as surfaces go, a running track is great, asphalt is better than concrete, and dirt or silt on the side of the road is best
- Stay safe – be aware of your surroundings. Run during the day or in well-lit places and run with a partner when you can
- Wear a watch so you can time your runs
- Record your runs in your fitness diary
- Land on heels and roll forward
- Keep your shoulders back
- Don't clench your fists
- Bend your elbows at the waist with hands facing each other, and keep your elbows close to your body and not out to the side
- Look straight ahead – don't stare down at your feet

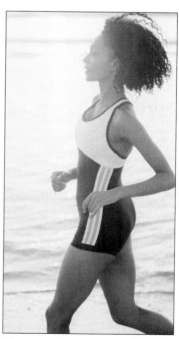

■ **Running is good** *cardiovascular exercise – but be patient at first and don't push yourself too hard.*

Don't forget to warm up, stretch, and cool down when you run or walk.

Sign up for a road race

A running programme is more likely to succeed if you have a concrete goal to aim for. Even seasoned athletes need that carrot dangling in front of them. That's why signing up for a 5k (5-kilometre or 3.1-mile) road race is a great goal for beginning runners and walkers.

Not only is running a road race an excellent goal, it's just plain fun. Most races have a wide variety of runners and walkers. It's great to hear people cheering on the sidelines, and to be with all those people with whom you share a common goal. There's nothing like running through that finish line – and most runs have free snacks and drinks once you finish.

If you're starting from scratch, or if you can't walk comfortably for an hour at a time, give yourself a few months to prepare. If you can walk for an hour with no problem, then you don't need quite that much lead time. Opposite is a sample 3-week training schedule to help you get ready for a 5k run. Remember that these are suggestions. You should always progress at your own pace. Even on race day, walking is always allowed. For the first race especially, getting through the finish line is the ultimate goal. Once you've mastered that, you can think about pushing up the speed and training a bit to keep it interesting.

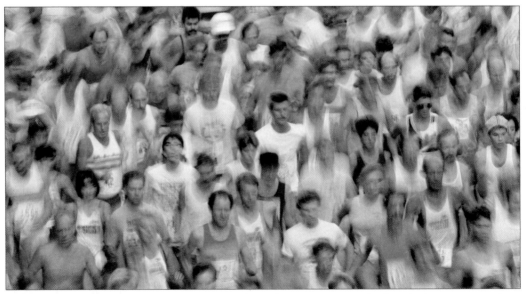

■ **Training for a road race** *will help keep you focused as you exercise. The fun of taking part in such an event and the satisfaction of going the distance are great motivators to spur you on still farther.*

Training schedule for a 5k (3.1-mile) run

Record your walks and runs in your fitness journal.

Don't move to the next day or week until you are totally comfortable with the level you're on. If that means repeating Sunday's 1.6 km (1-mile) walk all week, do that.

WEEK 1
Goal: *To jog 1.6 km (1 mile) without stopping*

Sunday:	1.6 km (1-mile) walk
Monday:	1.6 km (1-mile) walk and/or jog (begin to mix in light jogging)
Tuesday:	1.6 km (1-mile) walk and/or jog
Wednesday:	Rest
Thursday:	1.6 km (1-mile) jog. Try to jog the entire 1.5 km
Friday:	1.6 km (1-mile) jog
Saturday:	Rest

● *Stay on this routine until you feel comfortable jogging 1.6 km (1 mile)*

WEEK 2
Goal: *To increase your longest run to 3.2 km (2 miles)*

Sunday:	1.6 km (1-mile) nonstop jog, relaxed pace
Monday:	12-minute nonstop jog
Tuesday:	1.6 km (1-mile) nonstop run (if you're up to it, try going a bit faster)
Wednesday:	Rest
Thursday:	3.2 km (2-mile) walk and/or jog
Friday:	1.6 km (1-mile) nonstop jog, relaxed pace
Saturday:	Rest

● *Stay on this routine until you feel comfortable running 3 km (2 miles)*

WEEK 3
Goal: *Run for 5 km (3.1 miles)*

Sunday:	3.2 km (2-mile) jog, relaxed pace
Monday:	15-minute nonstop jog
Tuesday:	3.2 km (2-mile) nonstop jog (if you're up to it, try going a little faster)
Wednesday:	Rest
Thursday:	15-minute nonstop jog
Friday:	5 km (3.1-mile) jog
Saturday:	Rest

● *Congratulations! Once you've hit this milestone, you are ready for your 5k run*

Training schedule for a 10k (6.2-mile run)

If it's a 10k, or 6.2-mile run you're after, or if you just want to keep going, read on.

If you have access to a treadmill, you won't have to let bad weather keep you from running.

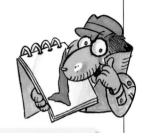

WEEK 4

Goal: *To run a fast 3.2 km (2 miles). How fast depends on athletic ability, age, and running experience. An average runner might try a 6–6.5 minutes per km (9–10 minutes per mile) pace.*

Sunday:	5 km (3.1-mile) jog
Monday:	15-minute relaxed jog
Tuesday:	3.2 km (2-mile) run (time yourself)
Wednesday:	Rest
Thursday:	10-minute *out and back run*
Friday:	15-minute relaxed jog
Saturday:	Rest

WEEK 5

Goal: *To run 6.4 km (4 miles) nonstop*

Sunday:	10-minute out and back run
Monday:	3.2 km (2-mile) relaxed jog
Tuesday:	3.2 km (2-mile) timed run (take the same route you timed last week and time it again)
Wednesday:	Rest
Thursday:	15-minute relaxed jog
Friday:	6.4 km (4-mile) jog
Saturday:	Rest

WEEK 6

Goal: *An 8 km (5-mile) nonstop run*

Sunday:	10-minute out and back run
Monday:	3.2 km (2-mile) relaxed jog
Tuesday:	4.8 km (3-mile) timed run (focus on running a quick, steady pace)
Wednesday:	Rest
Thursday:	15-minute relaxed jog
Friday:	8 km (5-mile) nonstop jog
Saturday:	Rest

> **DEFINITION**
>
> An **out and back run** is designed to improve your endurance for the second half of a race and teach you how to pace yourself through it. Run for 10 minutes at a brisk pace, then turn around and retrace your path home, aiming to get back in under 10 minutes.

WEEK 7
Goal: *A 10k (6.2 mile) nonstop run!*

Sunday:	15-minute out and back run
Monday:	3.2 km (2-mile) relaxed jog
Tuesday:	4.8 km (3-mile) timed run
Wednesday:	Rest
Thursday:	15-minute relaxed jog
Friday:	10 km (6.2-mile) nonstop run
Saturday:	Rest

WEEK 8
Goal: *To run 8 km (5 miles) at a steady pace*

Sunday:	8 km (5-mile) run at a relaxed pace
Monday:	15-minute relaxed jog
Tuesday:	15-minute out and back run
Wednesday:	Rest
Thursday:	8 km (5-mile) relaxed jog
Friday:	8 km (5-mile) timed run
Saturday:	Rest

Don't run hard the day or two before the race – conserve your energy.

WEEK 9
Goal: *To continue to build your endurance and prepare your body for race day*

Sunday:	8 km (5 miles) at race pace (this doesn't have to be super fast, just whatever speed you plan on going on race day)
Monday:	20-minute run at relaxed pace
Tuesday:	8 km (5-mile) run at relaxed pace
Wednesday:	20-minute run at relaxed pace
Thursday:	Rest
Friday:	20-minute run at relaxed pace
Saturday:	Rest
Sunday:	Race day – have fun!

● *Running through the finish line at any speed is something to be proud of. Even on race day, don't push yourself to injury just to get ahead. Go at your own speed and do your best.*

INTERNET

www.coolrunning.com/
major/97/training/5k/
glen0.htm

For more info on training for a 5k (3.1 miles) or 10k (6.2 miles), or if you want more running tips, click here.

Cycling

WHEN YOU WERE A CHILD, *did you ever just hop on your bike and ride around for no reason – or just to explore the neighbourhood or hang out with friends? Well, even if you didn't, it's never too late to start. Whether you live in an urban area, or out in the country, riding a bike is great aerobic exercise. It develops strength, stamina, and balance. Get in touch with your inner child! Hop on a bike and explore.*

Mountain bikes

Although mountain bikes, which hit the streets about 15 years ago, are the newest kids on the block, they've become the most popular. They're rugged and versatile, so they're great for trail riding and off-road excursions, but they can also be used on the road (although they are a little slower on pavement than are road bikes). Mountain bike tyres are fat and knobby. The seat is in an upright position, which many people find more comfortable than the stretched out riding position. The frames are made out of high-tech materials, and they're sturdy and lightweight.

A mountain bike is a good choice if you plan on hitting the trails. If you've never ridden on trails before, be careful. I've ridden bikes my whole life, but my first few times trying to stay on those skinny trails on a mountain bike were challenging! It's hard to stay steady over all those rocks, bumps, and curves if you're not used to it. Of course, the beautiful scenery more than made up for the difficulty.

When you're going downhill on a mountain bike, lean back into your seat. It's tempting to stand up and lean forward, but you might just topple over the handlebars. I found that out the hard way.

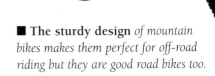

■ **The sturdy design** *of mountain bikes makes them perfect for off-road riding but they are good road bikes too.*

Cross bikes

Cross bikes are also called "hybrids" because they have some elements of mountain bikes and some of road bikes. While their tyres are thinner than those of mountain bikes, they're still wider than road bike tyres. Cross bikes have between 18 and 24 gears. These are great for fitness riding, city cycling, commuting, or even a little light trail riding.

Road bikes

The road bike is the traditional European road-racing bike. It's best for high-speed street riding. The road bike has skinny tyres and drop handlebars so that you ride in an aerodynamic, stretched-out position, and has between 12 and 21 gears. Don't go off road with this one; the tyres are too thin. The road bike is for training, triathlons, or long mileage.

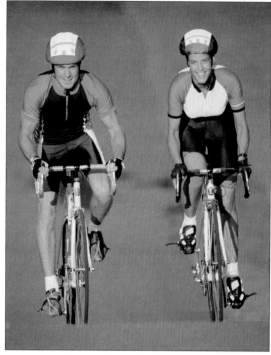

■ **Skinny tyres and drop handlebars** *make road bikes more aerodynamic than their off-road counterparts, so they're ideal for high-speed racing.*

Touring bikes

Touring bikes are built for the long haul. They're a bit like road bikes but are more durable and comfortable. They're good for extended trips because they're built to carry additional equipment. These have between 18 and 24 gears, and also have the drop handlebars.

Trivia...

Did he or didn't he? Leonardo da Vinci is often credited with sketching out the first bicycle design, but recent discoveries reveal that the materials used to make the drawing weren't invented until decades after his death.

Other bikes

There are also beach cruisers with big tyres, for easy rides along the shore. And there are general lightweights – single speed and three-speed bikes. These are good for trips to the store, or for a mellow ride to the neighbours, but if you go on a bike ride with friends who have bikes with more gears, you're going to be left behind on the hills.

Finally, there are also tandem bikes that are built for two, which can be fun.

Biking necessities

No matter what kind of cycling you're going to do, here's a list of must-haves:

- **Helmet**: this is the one thing you can't do without! Don't buy a bike without purchasing a helmet. I've seen someone without a helmet take the smallest spill, and yet she couldn't remember her name or where she was as we drove to the hospital. Wear a helmet!
- **Gloves**: these can help you keep your grip on the handlebars even if you get sweaty, but most importantly they can protect your palms if you take a tumble
- **Water bottle**: with any aerobic activity, it's important to stay hydrated. Always bring a bottle of water on your bike trips
- **Sunglasses**: these not only protect your eyes from the sun, they keep nasty bugs out

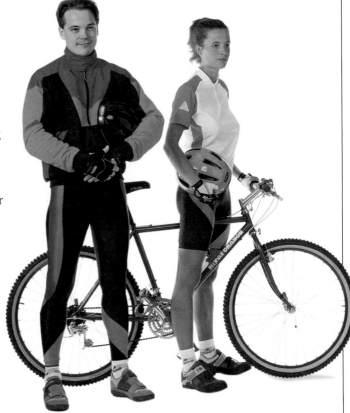

■ **Protective helmets and gloves** *are essential for preventing injury in the event of a fall. It's also important to wear comfortable shoes, and clothing that won't snag.*

Tips for bike workouts

The great thing about riding bikes is that you'll get better fast. Always start with a 10–15 minute warm-up and stretch. If you are a beginner, start with a relatively flat stretch where you can ride consistently for 5 minutes. After that, rev up to a speed so that you're in your target heart rate, and stay at that level for 10 minutes to start, gradually working up to 30–45 minutes. Keep this up for about 3 weeks, three times a week if you have time. After about 4–6 weeks, you can increase your distance and start adding some hills. Remember – the amount of time it takes to move up to the next level is different for everyone. If after 3 weeks you're not ready to increase distance or speed, then stay where you are for a little longer.

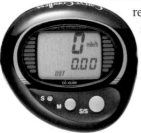

CYCLE COMPUTER

In the pool

SWIMMING IS ONE OF MY *favourite ways to stay in shape. It exercises the whole body – legs, arms, and back – without stressing the joints or muscles. Swimming is a wonderful option for people who are overweight, or who have joint or muscle problems, because they become weightless in the water. The benefit of being weightless is that there is no impact on the body, so you can get a workout that's just as effective as high-impact aerobics or running, minus the pain. You can still get sore, of course, but swimming is much easier on your body than many other aerobic activities.*

Take a lesson. Even if you're a great swimmer, a lesson can help improve your form and add renewed challenges to your swimming workout. I was in a swimming team for 15 years, and I was a lifeguard for years after that, but I recently took a lesson and learned a lot that improved my stroke. I had fallen into quite a few bad habits over the years and had no idea!

If you're just starting out, start slowly. Don't forget to warm up, stretch, and cool down. Start with any stroke – I've heard that backstroke burns the most calories – and go at your own pace, gradually working up to 30 minutes of continuous swimming.

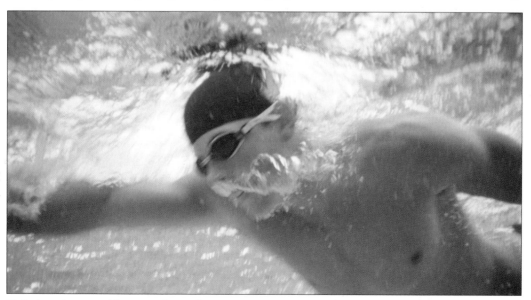

■ **Swimming provides a workout** *that's just as vigorous as aerobics or running – but because your body is supported by the water, it doesn't jar or strain your muscles and joints.*

Aerobics with a splash

Water aerobics is another way to exercise in the pool. Many gyms now offer a variety of water aerobics classes. I've even taken an "underwater kickboxing" class. These classes are great for older adults, for people who are rehabilitating injuries, or for anyone who just wants a pleasant, safe workout. Even if you're in great shape, water aerobics can be a fun addition to your lap swim. Tips you learn in water aerobics classes can enrich anyone's experience in the pool.

Between laps, I often like to use this move I learned in a water aerobics class: hold onto the side of the pool with one hand, and trace the alphabet with your right toe on the bottom. In other words, pretend that you're writing the alphabet on the bottom of the pool with your toe. When you get to Z, change sides and do it with the left foot. It gives your leg muscles an extra dose of toning.

Team sports

JOINING A TEAM CAN GIVE *your workout a boost. For one thing, playing a game gets your mind off the fact that you're burning calories. If you like camaraderie and competition, join a team! You could join a local league, gather a group of friends, or get a group from work together to vent some frustrations on the field.*

Football, rugby, netball, and hockey are all great aerobic workouts, while rounders and volleyball are less rigorous. Any game in which you're standing around a lot waiting for the ball is less of an aerobic workout. That just means you might add a jog around the field to your games.

In the US, Ultimate Frisbee is a team sport that is rapidly gaining in popularity. It's similar to football, and provides a great aerobic workout. The best thing about it is that all that's really needed is a Frisbee and a field (and seven people on each side).

Before you join a team, check it out. Some teams just want to get out there and have fun while others are out to win, win, win! Think about what you want – a highly competitive game where the best players get most of the on-field time, or a more

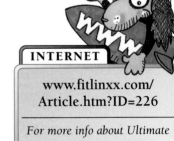

INTERNET

www.fitlinxx.com/
Article.htm?ID=226

For more info about Ultimate Frisbee, including a training guide, log on here.

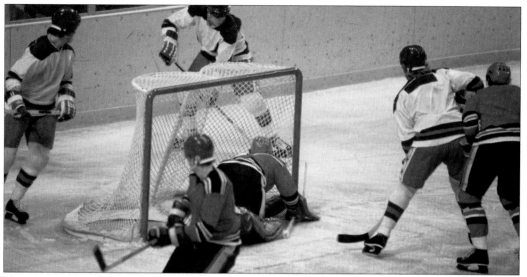

■ **Many team sports,** *such as ice hockey, provide a vigorous aerobic workout. As part of a competitive team, focusing on the game also helps take your mind off how much you're exerting yourself.*

fun atmosphere where everyone plays. Everyone is different. If you prefer to exercise solo and compete only with yourself, perhaps running or swimming might be a better option. If you're not sure, try everything! You may discover skills and interests you didn't even know you had.

A simple summary

✔ The exact number of calories you burn with each activity is affected by many variables.

✔ Fitness walking can be an exercise unto itself or a lead-in to running.

✔ Signing up to run in a road race can give your running workout a jump-start.

✔ There are all kinds of bikes out there – find one you like and hop on.

✔ Swimming laps isn't the only way to get in shape in the pool. Try water aerobics.

✔ Joining a team might entice you to put more energy into your workout.

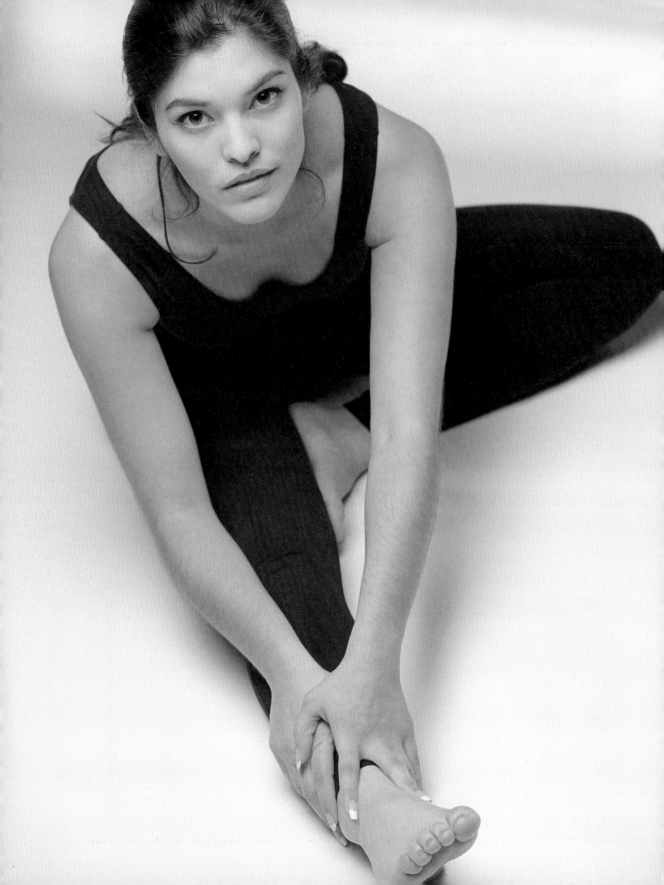

Chapter 9

Lengthen and Strengthen

HOW CAN YOU GET LONG AND LEAN? Let us count the ways. There are Eastern disciplines such as yoga and tai chi that forge the mind-body connection and help you loosen up and get supple. There are also Pilates and Lotte Berk, methods designed to bring awareness to the body and help you become taut and lean. Then there's classical ballet dancing that produces the most lithe, graceful bodies. And last but not least – in-line skating, which is a popular way to tone up while you're out having fun. In this chapter, we'll go through the basics of all the exercise disciplines above. I'll give you the lowdown on yoga, tai chi, Pilates, and Lotte Berk, and I've thrown in a few moves for you to try at home.

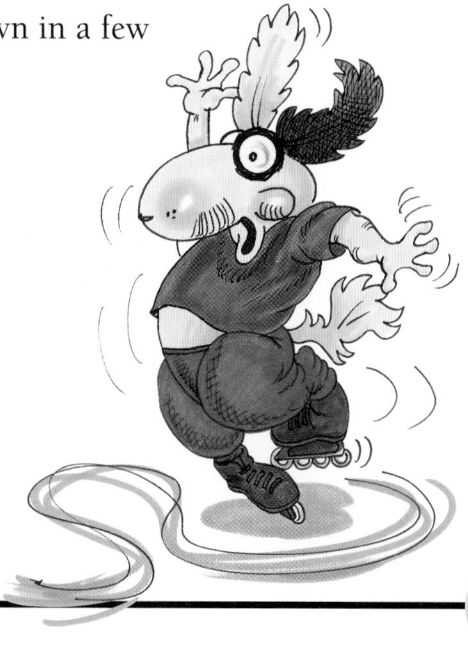

✓ **Eastern influence**

✓ **Low-impact stretching and toning methods**

✓ **In-line skating**

STRETCHING PROMOTES FLEXIBILITY AND SUPPLENESS

Eastern influence

AS PEOPLE LOOK FOR ALTERNATIVE WAYS to get healthy, Eastern disciplines such as yoga and tai chi are growing increasingly popular. In addition to specialized studios, more gyms offer these classes along with their regular aerobic fare. Yoga and tai chi are both disciplines that unite the mind and body.

Yoga

Yoga can be a great way to relieve stress and get a workout. It cultivates cardiovascular health, strength, and flexibility. It also tunes up your organs. Many people who do a lot of yoga say that it's the only exercise they need to stay in great shape. I prefer to mix yoga into my routine as a stretching, meditative exercise and continue doing other activities for cardio and strength training.

Stretching, along with aerobic activity and strength training, makes up a complete exercise programme.

Of course, how much supplementary exercise you need has a lot to do with what level your yoga practice is on. Some types of yoga are more physically challenging than others. In general, yoga is a slow, meditative stretch that links the mind and body. Yoga literally means "union".

The best way to learn yoga is by taking a class. At the beginning of a yoga class, you grab a mat and sit down on the floor. Then the instructor will often chant "oomm" with the class. Next begins the series of postures, or *asanas*. The postures in yoga are held for a long time as you breathe deeply and relax further into the posture. Being aware of your breath is a vital aspect of yoga.

> ### Trivia...
> Yoga began as a spiritual discipline in India as far back as 1800 BC. These days, more than 500,000 people in the UK do yoga on a regular basis.

> **DEFINITION**
>
> **Asanas** *are the physical postures of yoga.*

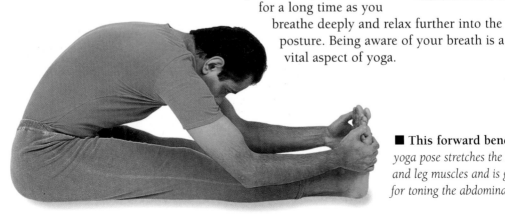

■ **This forward bending** *yoga pose stretches the back and leg muscles and is good for toning the abdominal area.*

Tips for taking your first yoga class

- Wear loose clothes that you can move around in comfortably
- Be prepared to be barefoot
- Don't compare yourself to people around you; go as far into the postures as *you* can
- Find a teacher with a soothing voice, someone whose voice you like; this person will be guiding you through the postures

The first time I went to a yoga class, I was sceptical. I thought, "Well, I do want to relax and stretch, but I can't take this seriously. There's no way I'm saying 'oomm'." Gradually, though, I relaxed my mind and body and came to really enjoy practising yoga.

Now that I've taken a few yoga classes, I find that I incorporate some of the asanas in my stretching routine before other activities. I notice a lot of similarities in the moves, too, during stretching sessions of some aerobic, dance, or even toning classes. I've noticed many athletes using yoga-inspired stretches, too.

Don't hold your breath while you do yoga. Your breath should be deep and natural.

One of the first yoga exercises I learned, and one that I continue to do, is called "Sun Salutation", and it's a series of 12 poses. Turn the page and you'll find out how to do it. Take your time and stay in each position for as long as you need to. If one pose feels particularly good, stay there longer. Breathe deeply. Each position should flow smoothly into the next.

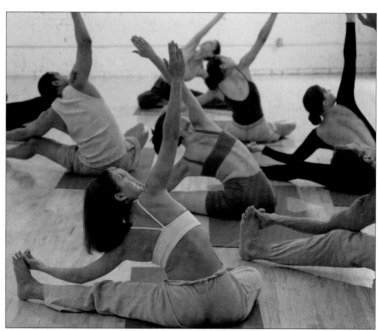

■ **In addition to the** *different styles and schools of yoga, there are many variations and interpretations, depending on the teacher you choose. What's important is to choose a teacher you resonate with, no matter what their style.*

SUN SALUTATION

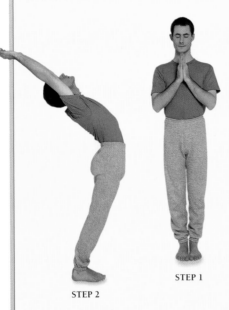

1 Stand with your feet together, shoulders down and relaxed. Press your palms together in front of your heart.

2 Raise your arms (with palms still together) over and behind your head. Lean your head back and open up your chest and palms.

3 Bring your arms back down, keeping them straight out in front of you. With a flat back, bend all the way over until your palms are on the floor (or as close as they come). Bring your nose and chest towards your knees.

4 If your palms aren't on the floor, bend your knees until they are. Place your left foot between your hands, knee bent, and stretch your right leg out behind you. Look straight ahead.

5 Bring your left foot back to meet the right, and straighten out your body so that you're in the plank pose, as if you were at the top of a push-up. Keep your shoulders relaxed, and breathe.

6 Lower your body down to the floor so that your chest is on the floor, keeping your weight on your hands. Keep a slight bend in the middle.

STEP 1

STEP 2

STEP 3

STEP 4

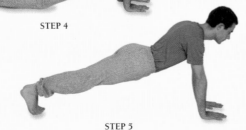

STEP 5

STEP 6

7 Raise your head up like a snake, arching your back and opening your chest.

8 Bring your head back down and lift up again so that you're in the triangle pose.

9 Now bring your right foot between your hands and stretch your left leg out behind you. Lift your head up.

10 Step your left foot forwards to meet the right, bend over with your legs straight (but don't lock your knees). Let your head hang over your knees. Try to bring your chest close to your legs.

11 Leading with your arms out in front, and keeping your back flat, rise up to a standing position. Keep going all the way back. With your arms above your head, lean your head back and open up your chest.

12 Bring your head and arms back, and press your palms together in front of your chest.

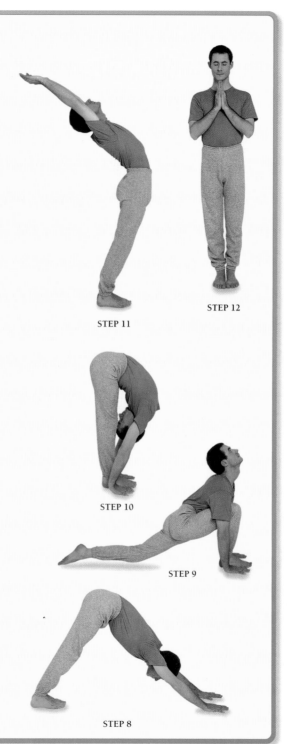

STEP 11

STEP 12

STEP 10

STEP 9

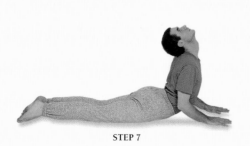

STEP 7

STEP 8

Tai chi

This ancient practice can help if you're feeling pressurized and stressed, out of balance, or just need to get focused.

T'ai chi chu'an (usually abbreviated to tai chi) is a centuries-old Chinese discipline. It's a moving meditation that can put the fire back in your eyes by moving energy through your body, increasing the flow of chi, or life force.

The exercise is a series of bending, stretching, twisting, and breathing patterns that uses movement and stillness to create body awareness and to calm internal energy. It's a great way to simultaneously relax and sharpen your focus, and it's best done outside. Maybe you've seen people in the park, moving very slowly, concentrating deeply. Chances are, they were doing tai chi.

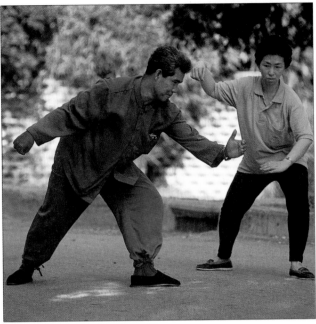

■ **Tai chi** *is one of the most popular exercise systems in the world – it is practised by millions of people every day.*

Learning the form

As a low-impact and low-intensity activity, tai chi benefits everyone; it's especially good for older adults or for people recovering from injuries. The physical and mental benefits are vast. Tai chi can increase balance, relieve stress, improve concentration, circulation, and posture, and give a general sense of wellbeing.

Tai chi exercises consist of a set of forms. Each form consists of a series of positions that are strung together in one continuous movement. Forms vary; a single form can contain up to 100 positions and could take as long as 20 minutes to complete. The average form takes about 7–10 minutes.

The forms on the following pages can take anywhere from 5–10 minutes each. They shouldn't be rushed. Wear comfortable, loose-fitting clothes and flat shoes, socks, or bare feet. Tai chi can be done any time, anywhere, but it's recommended that you do it the same time every day for maximum benefits. The goal is to achieve a balanced stillness in the mind while taking the body through fluid, co-ordinated movements.

*The **tantien** is the area just below the navel. It's considered the centre of the body's chi. In Chinese philosophy, chi is the life force, or vital energy. Tai chi aims to sink the chi back into the tantien; the chi floats up to the head and upper torso when we get stressed. Tai chi helps release chi, allowing it to move freely through your body. Chinese medicine assumes that blocked chi causes discomfort, illness, and disease.*

When doing tai chi, knees should remain slightly bent, and all movement should originate from the **tantien.** Breathing should be slow, deep, and natural; never force your breath. Here are a few basic tai chi exercises. There are different types of tai chi, based on the family each originated from. These exercises are from the Wu family.

General stance

When standing, your feet should be parallel and shoulder-width apart, and your knees should be loose and relaxed. Release your pelvis so that your tailbone points to the ground, opening up the lumbar region.

Lift your spine, keeping your head aligned directly over your spine (not forwards, back, or to the side). Let your shoulder blades sink towards your hips. Relax your chest so that you can feel your breath down into your belly.

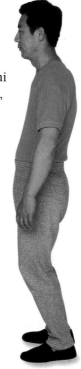

GENERAL STANCE

Four forms

Each form consists of various positions that should flow smoothly into each other. The movements should be soft, without any stress or discomfort.

Commencement form:

1 Stand with your arms by your sides, palms facing back

2 Raise arms and bend elbows in towards your waist; then circle back down to starting position

3 Raise arms straight out in front of you (without locking elbows), keeping hands relaxed and palms facing the ground

4 Lower arms slowly down, keeping palms parallel to the ground

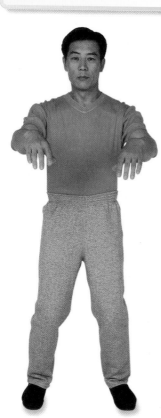

COMMENCEMENT FORM

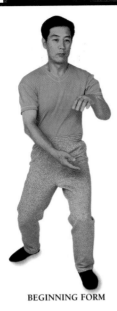

BEGINNING FORM

Beginning form:

5. Turn hands out, so fingertips point away from body. Keep elbows bent and close to sides

6. Bring arms in front of your chest, with your right hand lower, palm out, and your left hand higher, with the palm facing in. Put your left foot forwards, and keep your weight on the right foot. Keeping your elbows down, circle your hands in front of you, keeping the movement steady and calm

7. Turn your body to the right. Step right foot forwards and shift weight to left foot. With right palm up, touch left fingertips to the right wrist

Grasp the bird's tail form:

8. Bend knees and turn to the left. Turn right palm in, keeping left fingertips at wrist

9. Shift weight forwards and turn to the right

10. Continue turning to the right until you have made a complete circle, returning to centre

GRASP THE BIRD'S TAIL

11. Shift weight to the right and turn to the left. Change the position of your hands – right palm faces away from the body and left palm faces body, still touching at the pulse

Single whip:

12. Bend right wrist over left hand, bringing the right fingers and thumb together, pointing down. Then turn left palm towards body (fingers still at right wrist), and take a small step back with left foot. With your right arm steady and weight on right leg, move left foot back to centre

13. Move each arm out to the side, keeping shoulders down. Keep fingers and thumbs of right hand together and pointing down, while left palm faces out. Each wrist should be at shoulder height, elbows bent towards ground, with weight distributed equally on each leg

SINGLE WHIP

Low-impact stretching and toning methods

THERE ARE ALSO MANY LOW-IMPACT *stretching and toning methods that come from the West. More recently developed exercise disciplines include Pilates and the Lotte Berk method, named after the people who developed them, Joseph Pilates and Lotte Berk, who were life-long champions of physical fitness. Both methods can be used as a workout, as a stretching and toning supplement, or even for rehabilitation because all the movements are low-impact (no jumping or other jarring movements) and many can be done while lying down.*

These exercises are great if you're rehabilitating from an injury or if you have a physical disability. The Pilates regimen sprang from Joseph Pilates' determination to strengthen his frail and sickly body (he had asthma and rickets as a child), and Lotte Berk developed her exercises after experiencing a debilitating back injury. Photos of Joseph Pilates at age 70 reveal a slim, toned physique, and Lotte Berk also remained lithe and youthful into old age.

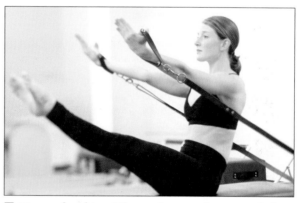

■ **It's worth taking Pilates classes** *to learn exactly how to do the moves, because positioning is very important.*

Pilates

Pronounced "pi-lah-tees", this 90-year-old exercise discipline can improve your posture, help you get long, lean muscles, and tighten those abs. It also gets the blood circulating and improves balance. Joseph Pilates began developing his method of strengthening and stretching he called "the Art of Controlology" in Germany in the 1900s.

Most Pilates moves can be done on a mat, but there is also specialized equipment you can use at a Pilates studio.

Trivia...
Interned during World War I, Joseph Pilates taught his mat work to everyone in his barracks. During an influenza outbreak, they were the only people who didn't get sick.

147

There are many books and videos on Pilates, but I recommend taking a class or two. Take a one-on-one class if you can, because it's very helpful to have someone show you exactly how to do the moves. It's all about subtle positioning and controlling your body.

The Pilates Body by Brooke Siler is an excellent resource for Pilates. It's got detailed descriptions of the mat work and covers a bit of Pilates history. In the meantime, here's a little sample. Get a mat or towel and get down on the floor for some Pilates mat moves. In Pilates, the movements come from your *powerhouse*.

DEFINITION

Your **powerhouse** *is the area just below your belt line.*

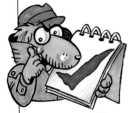

The "Hundred"

Here's a basic Pilates mat move to get you started.

I find that if I do the "Hundred" first thing in the morning, it really helps wake me up.

1 Lie on your back and pull your knees into your chest. Inhale deeply, and as you exhale, sink your chest and belly into the mat beneath you

2 Press your torso down as you bring your head up and face your belly. Lift with your upper back, not your neck, until you feel the bottom of your shoulder blades pressing into the mat

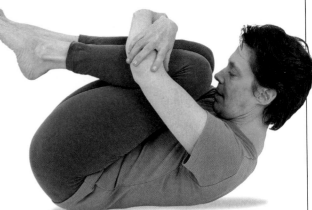

STEP 1

3 Straighten your legs up, squeezing your rear and inner thighs together. For the first few times, keep your legs up at a 90-degree angle. As you get better, you can lower your legs to eye level

4 Once you're in position, stretch your arms out from your sides as if you were trying to touch the wall across the room with your fingertips. Now, pump your arms straight up and down as if you were slapping water for 100 counts. Inhale for five counts, and exhale for five, and so on until you get to 100

Lotte Berk method

Like Pilates, the Lotte Berk method, or just Lotte Berk, is named after the person who created it. The method involves some of the same principles of getting tuned into your body and of using small, controlled movements to develop a long, lithe look.

The famous modern dancer, Lotte Berk, created this method in Germany in the 1970s. After she suffered a back injury, she developed it to help her stay fit and supple without the use of equipment or machines. Now the method is used to help people develop the long, taut look of a dancer. The body position for Lotte Berk is strict alignment, with the pelvis tucked forward. Here are some moves from the Lotte Berk method to get you started:

INTERNET

www.lotteberk.ch

For more on Lotte Berk, including glamorous photos of the dancer, go to this web site for the Lotte Berk studio in Zurich. Although most of it is in German, there's a great quote from her in English.

Warm-up: marching

Stand up nice and tall, and lift your knees to your chest as you swing your arms out in the opposite direction. Keep your toes pointed down when you lift your knee, and keep your feet close to your body. Keep your arms straight. Do this 100 times.

All Lotte Berk movements should be controlled. Remember to keep your pelvis tucked forwards.

Standing seat exercise

(In Lotte Berk, the rear end is called the seat.)

1. Standing with your pelvis tucked in and your abs in, hold on to something sturdy like a wall, and place your right leg back behind you. Point your right toe, and keep your right leg straight

2. Lift right leg several centimetres off the ground while maintaining straight posture. Lift right leg up in small movements 20 times and then switch legs

Back dancing

3. Lie down on a mat or towel with your knees slightly bent and your feet flat on the floor

4. Tuck your pelvis under and raise hips several centimetres from the mat. Pulse up for 2 minutes, rest, and repeat

WALK LIKE A DANCER

Have you ever seen a ballet dancer with bad posture? They might exist, but I've never seen one. Most ballet dancers stand tall. While practising ballet isn't going to make you any taller, it can make you stand taller and develop elongated muscles.

It would be impossible for me to train you for the Bolshoi by book, but I can pass along some ballet tips that you can incorporate into your exercise to help you get those long, lean features and stand taller.

Here are the five basic ballet positions of the feet to help you move like a graceful swan. Just practising these positions – while standing up straight, tightening your leg muscles, and holding in your stomach – can improve your posture and increase body-awareness.

Try these moves at home or even while you're waiting for the bus or standing on the station platform.

Every step of movement in ballet originates from one of these five basic positions.

■ **Practising ballet moves** *can help you improve muscle tone and posture so that you stand taller and move more gracefully.*

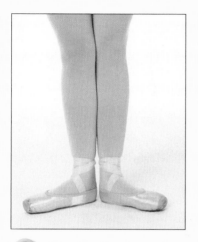

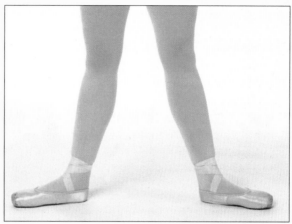

1 **First position:**

Point toes out so that feet form one line, heels touching.

2 **Second position:**

The feet are on the same line but with a distance of about 30 cm (1 foot) between the heels.

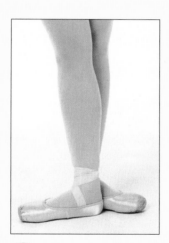

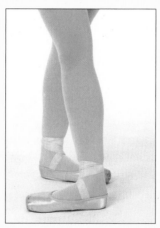

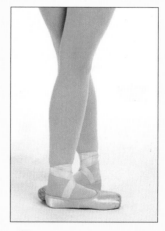

3 **Third position:**

Place one foot in front of the other, heel touching the middle of the other foot.

4 **Fourth position:**

Place the feet so that they are parallel and separated by the length of one foot.

5 **Fifth position:**

Cross the feet so that the first joint of the big toe shows beyond each heel.

In-line skating

"WHAT'S IN-LINE SKATING DOING with all these stretching techniques?" you might ask. Well, besides giving a great aerobic workout, in-line skating also helps you get long and lean legs and tones your rear in no time.

In-line skates were first invented in the 1700s by a Dutchman who wanted to simulate ice skating in the summer. Over 200 years later, in-line skating has spread from its modern roots in the US right around the world.

In-line skating is one of the best forms of exercise for toning the muscles in your legs and buttocks. It burns about 400 calories an hour, but is less stressful on your joints and organs than high-impact exercises like running (unless, of course, you fall a lot). It's a great aerobic exercise because you can get your heart rate up for a long time.

In-line skating helps tone your core body, because your abs and back are engaged even when you're just standing there balancing on skates.

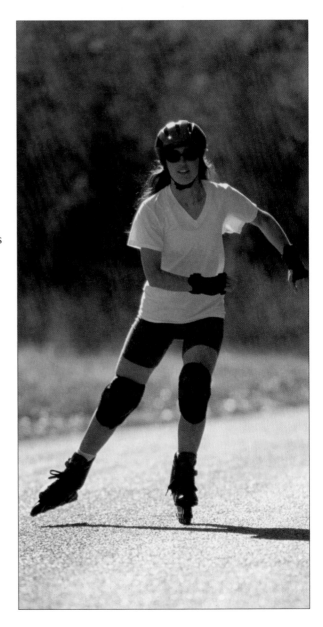

■ **In-line skating** *is so much fun that it hardly feels like exercise, but it's excellent for toning your legs and buttocks.*

Tips for beginners

Here are some tips on what to do, and what not to do, if you're a novice in-line skater. Read this before you hit the road.

Choose skates wisely

Rent or borrow skates before you buy. In-line skates can cost anywhere from £20 to £200, but you should expect to spend at least £70 for a quality pair. Start with a low-grade bearing (the grade of the ball bearings inside the wheels controls the speed of the skate). The lower the grade, the slower the skate; and that's a good thing for beginners. Speedy, high-grade bearings are harder to control, especially when stepping up on a kerb or going downhill. Once you get the hang of the low-grade bearings, you can move up.

Get kitted out!

You may feel like a Robo-person with a helmet and knee, elbow, and wrist pads, but you need all of these. You're more likely to be aggressive and learn faster if you have the sense of security that comes from being protected.

You can pare down a little once you're sure-footed, but always wear a helmet. In addition to sprains and fractures, if you don't wear protective gear you're also a lot more vulnerable to scrapes, wrist, knee, or elbow dislocations, or even a serious head injury.

Don't forget to stretch — both before and after a skating session.

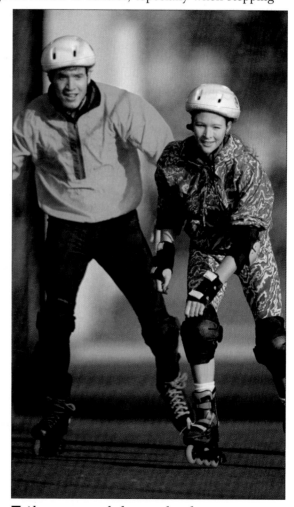

Don't work out cold muscles

Pulls or sprains are more likely if muscles are cold.

■ **Always wear a helmet and pads** *to protect yourself against wrist sprains and fractures, which are the most common injuries to in-line skaters.*

Things to remember when you're on the road

Here are a few important pointers to help keep you safe once you hit the streets.

Start in a safe area

Choose a smooth, flat, car-free site, such as an empty car park, a park, or a rink for in-line skating. Don't tempt fate by hitting the busy roads first. When you're on the streets, everything is magnified. Wait until you can manoeuvre quickly and confidently before you try crowded roads.

Push off gently from the side

Push off along the inside edge of your wheels. Keep your knees bent and your arms close to your body. Once you push off, your skate should go out to the side and not behind you.

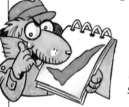

Keep your feet as close together as possible. When gliding, keep one foot slightly in front.

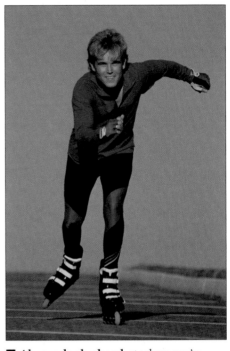

■ **Always look ahead** *at where you're going so that you can see curbs or rough spots and decide whether you want to avoid or negotiate them.*

Step on curbs or over rough spots

Keeping your feet close together, step up gently, one foot at a time.

Turn with your shoulders

Don't turn with your skates only. Instead, turn your shoulders in the direction you want to go, and your body will follow. Take it slowly at first, and once you're comfortable turning with your shoulders, you can move up to faster turns.

Don't pick up your feet

Don't move as if you were running or walking with a heel-to-toe movement. Also, don't smash your skates down. That could make them slide right out from under you.

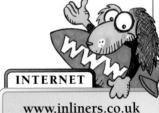

INTERNET

www.inliners.co.uk

Click here to find out more about in-line skating, and for directories of instructors and skating parks.

IN-LINE SKATING WORKOUT FOR NOVICES

Try the following workout a few times a week:

- Warm up for 5–10 minutes by walking briskly, jogging, or skating
- Stretch (see page 156)
- Practise balancing on skates on grass or some other soft surface. Balance on one skate for a few seconds and then try the other leg
- Start skating. With in-line skating, you can always glide, but you get a better workout when your feet are moving. Keep your feet moving for at least 2–3 minutes at a time at first; then work up to more
- To really work your legs, try holding a squat position. With weight centred over hips and arms out in front, bend knees as far as you can while keeping your balance. Add this to your regular skate and really feel the burn
- Start gradually and work up to skating for 40 minutes to an hour each session

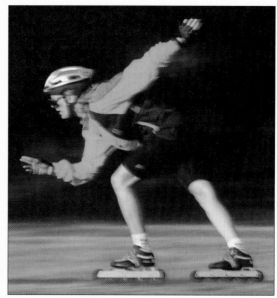

■ **To get the best workout** *you need to keep your feet moving and avoid too much gliding.*

Don't let your feet drift more than shoulder-width apart

This could cause you to lose control and you are more likely to fall.

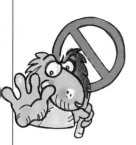

Don't lose concentration and blindly step on to a kerb or over something with your legs wide apart. You could end up doing the splits.

SEVEN STRETCHES FOR IN-LINE SKATING

1 While standing, lace fingers together, palms up, behind back. Push the inside of your elbows out and hold for 15 seconds

2 Stand with feet shoulder-width apart. Bring left elbow up and place hand behind right shoulder. Grab your left elbow with right hand and pull body gently to right side. Hold for 10 seconds and repeat on other side

3 Stand with feet shoulder-width apart. Put your hands on hips, keep back straight, and bend knees. Keep heels flat on floor. Hold for 30 seconds

4 Lean against a wall with your left leg bent and your right leg straight out behind. Keep your right heel flat on the ground. Hold for 15 seconds and change legs

5 Kneel down with your right leg in front and your left knee on the floor behind you. Place your hands on your right knee and extend left leg behind you so that you feel a stretch in your thigh. Hold for 15 seconds and repeat on other side

6 Sit down and place feet, soles together, in front of you. Hold your feet with your hands and gently push your knees down. Hold for 15–20 seconds

7 Sitting, extend your right leg in front and bend your left knee so that your left foot is on your inside right thigh. Reach for your right ankle with both hands, holding at the shin or ankle, wherever you feel the stretch without strain. Make sure your right knee stays straight and never bounces. Hold for 15–20 seconds and repeat on other side

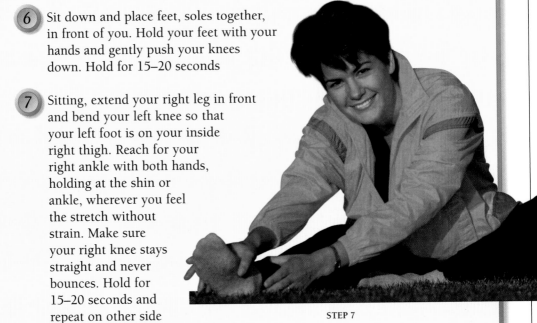

STEP 7

How to stop skating without killing yourself

It's not a good idea to rely on trees and stop signs to stop (ha) or to expect to screech to a halt. Give yourself about 4.5 metres (15 feet) to come to a stop. Here are some more tips.

Bend your knees

Hold your arms in front of your body, palms down. Keep your weight over your hips, move the brake skate out in front, lift your toe, and lower your hips as if doing a squat. When you feel the brake engage, continue to squat and apply pressure on the heel.

Practise falling

When you feel yourself starting to fall, crouch down – you'll have a shorter distance to fall – and fall forwards into your knee and wrist pads.

Avoid danger

Stay on smooth, dry surfaces. If you see a hill or other situation that looks dangerous, sit down, take your skates off, and walk. Don't approach a dangerous situation with your eyes closed and your fingers crossed.

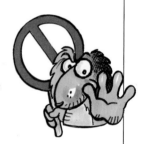

Don't flail your arms around. You're only making it harder to balance and further to fall.

Don't skate through water or sand

These can damage the bearings and affect skate performance.

A simple summary

✔ Yoga and tai chi can help you get supple and raise body awareness.

✔ Pilates and Lotte Berk are two popular alternatives to stretching. They incorporate dance-like stretches and fluid movements to help you get lithe and strong.

✔ Ballet dancers don't slump. Try the five basic ballet foot positions in your everyday life.

✔ In-line skating is a great way to develop long, lean muscles.

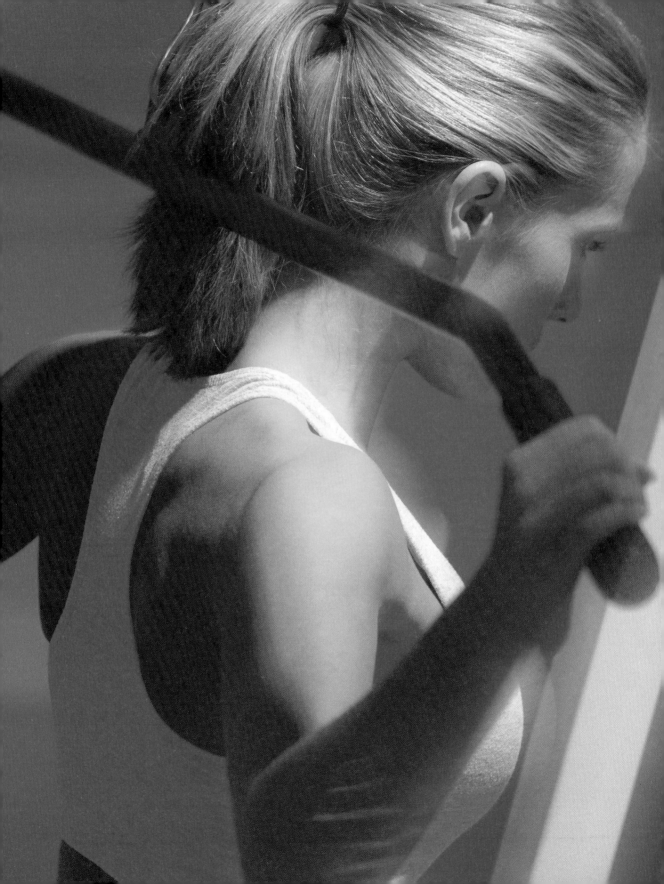

Chapter 10

Weight Training

N O WELL-ROUNDED FITNESS ROUTINE is complete without strength training, or working muscles against a resistance, such as weights. Learn about muscles – what they do and how to make them stronger without becoming the Incredible Hulk. You can get the results you want from a weight-training programme. There are many health benefits to being toned. With muscle strengthening, you can increase your bone density, become more powerful, and remain independent into old age.

In this chapter...

✔ Muscle know-how

✔ Why weight train?

✔ Work with your body type

✔ Rest builds muscle

✔ Get results

✔ Form is everything

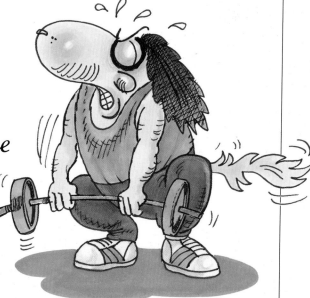

A WELL-DEFINED BODY IS JUST ONE BENEFIT OF WEIGHT TRAINING

Muscle know-how

THE HUMAN BODY IS A COMPLEX WEB *of bones, muscles, fat, skin, and so on. Muscles cover ligaments, bones, and joints and provide shape to the skeletal frame. While there are limitations to how much you can alter your shape, toning your muscles does affect the shape of your body. Larger muscles are near the surface of the body while smaller muscles tend to be deeper in the body. When exercising it's important to stretch and strengthen all the muscles through their full range of motion. Otherwise, shortening of the deeper muscles can occur and cause the stiffness we start to feel as we age. Regular stretching and strengthening can help. Muscles, tendons, and bones must all be healthy and functioning properly for the body to move normally.*

There are three types of muscles: smooth muscles that line the walls of internal organs (excluding the heart) and work involuntarily; cardiac muscles that work around the heart, also without conscious control; and finally skeletal muscles, the voluntary movement muscles that we'll concern ourselves with here.

Trivia...

There are over 450 muscles in the human body, and muscles make up at least 40 per cent of your body weight.

The skeletal muscles

Skeletal muscles, which are responsible for posture and movement, are attached to bones and are arranged in opposing groups around joints, such as those in the legs, back, and arms. For example, muscles that bend the elbow (biceps) are countered by muscles that straighten it (triceps). Whenever you do any weight training, you should work opposing muscle groups. We'll go into more detail about working opposing muscle groups a bit later on. Also, whenever you weight train, you should concentrate not only on the *concentric* contraction, which usually occurs during the lifting, but also concentrate on the *eccentric* contraction, which occurs as you're returning the weight to the starting point.

DEFINITION

When two ends of a muscle are brought together, it's a **concentric** *contraction. When two ends of a muscle move apart, it's called an* **eccentric** *contraction. When the length of the muscle doesn't alter but the muscle itself is placed against a resistance, as in arm wrestling, the contraction is called an isometric contraction.*

There is much talk these days about slow-twitch and fast-twitch muscle fibres and how these relate to training. Muscles are bundles of fibres that can contract. Basically, muscles are composed of two types of fibres – slow and fast twitch.

MUSCLE CHART

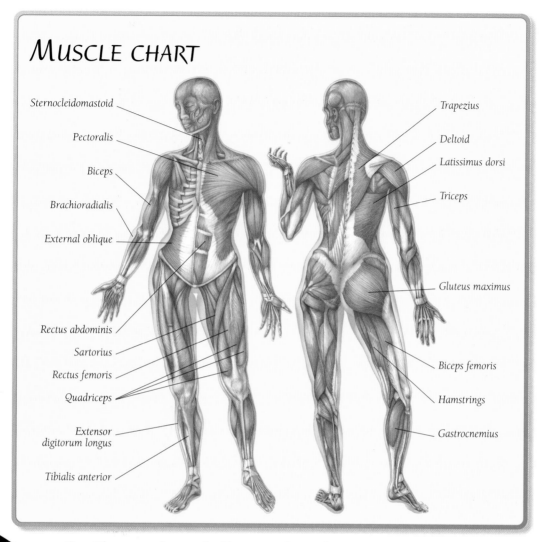

Sternocleidomastoid

Pectoralis

Biceps

Brachioradialis

External oblique

Rectus abdominis

Sartorius

Rectus femoris

Quadriceps

Extensor digitorum longus

Tibialis anterior

Trapezius

Deltoid

Latissimus dorsi

Triceps

Gluteus maximus

Biceps femoris

Hamstrings

Gastrocnemius

Slow-twitch muscle fibres are those that contract more slowly, are heartier (don't fatigue as easily), and are mostly used in endurance exercises. Fast-twitch muscle fibres contract quickly and are involved in quick movements. Most people have more of one kind or the other.

The balance of slow and fast twitch affects an individual's choice of activity in training. A person who has more slow-twitch muscles would be more inclined to long-distance running or to lifting weights for long periods, for example.

A person with more fast-twitch muscles would probably enjoy sprinting and choose to lift weights in short powerful bursts. It's something to think about when finding exercises you enjoy.

Why weight train?

ALONG WITH THE OTHER BENEFITS *of getting in shape – increased self-confidence, improved mood, longevity, and health – weight training has benefits of its own. While looking good in a bathing suit is great, there are even more reasons to get toned.*

Lifting weights builds muscles that can help you lose weight. Muscles burn more calories than fat because muscle is more metabolically active than fat, even when you're standing around and even while you sleep. In short, muscles are calorie-hungry in general and at all times burn more calories than does fat. Keep in mind, though, that if it's rapid weight loss you're after, cardio exercise is still your best bet.

The benefits of building strong bones

Weight-bearing exercise increases bone density. This is especially important as we get older because bone density, which increases until we're about 30 years old, begins to decrease after that age.

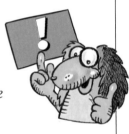

Weight-bearing exercise helps prevent osteoporosis, a progressive decrease in bone density that weakens bones and makes them more likely to fracture.

It's much easier to prevent osteoporosis than it is to treat it. This disease affects millions of people, especially older women. If you are a healthy male, however, do not skip over this section. Twenty per cent of the victims of osteoporosis are men. And if you're an older adult, strength training can help you remain independent. As you get stronger, you increase your ability to move around and reduce your chances of falling. Also, building bone density helps prevent hip and spinal fractures and other problems that can develop with age.

INTERNET

www.indiana.edu/~
health/weightrn/html

This US site has lots of information on the benefits of weight training plus helpful tips for beginners.

Improved posture

Strong back muscles lead to better posture and fewer lower back problems. Muscle building increases power and strength, making you more confident in all aspects of your life.

Many athletes include weight training in their fitness routine to improve their performance in other sports and to build strength that prevents their chances of injury.

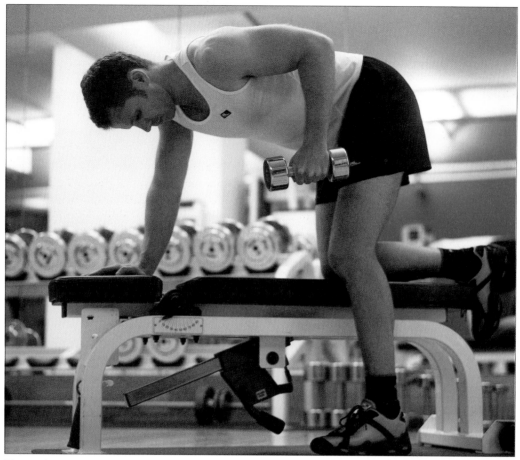

■ **Weight training builds strength and stamina.** *It also helps to increase bone density, so people who train regularly are less likely to suffer from fractures or other bone problems associated with aging.*

This means you may find marathoners sharing the weight room with you. Weight training is also a great way to stay in shape in the off season. Weight training for sports is most beneficial to performance when the intensity and movement closely resemble those of the sport. This means that even though they'll tone from head to toe, baseball players will work the muscles in their arms more vigorously, while football players will concentrate on their legs. Weight training is common among athletes from every kind of sport – baseball and football players, runners, dancers, and even racing drivers.

A water skier I know lifts weights to keep her body strong, not so much for the actual water skiing but so that she doesn't get hurt as badly when she falls. She likes to keep her body strong so it will stay in one piece.

Work with your body type

THE BAD NEWS FOR MEN *is that you're probably not going to bulk up like Arnold Schwarzenegger overnight or maybe ever. The good news for women is that you're probably not going to bulk up like Schwarzenegger overnight or maybe ever. In other words, your body is unique and will respond to weight training in its own way. Men tend to bulk up and women don't, but most women wouldn't aspire to Arnie's shape anyway. Also, keep in mind that many of the huge, ripped body builders you see take dangerous steroids and other drugs to pump up. Let's stay away from all that and get in shape the natural way.*

Every body responds differently to weight training.

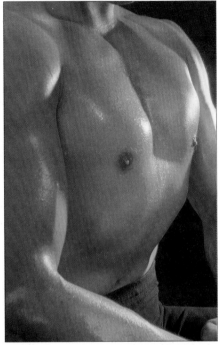

■ **Body builders** *may use unnatural means to build huge muscles.*

Women and men

Sometimes women hesitate to weight train because they don't want to get big, bulky muscles. The truth is that it's very hard for women to develop those bulging biceps because the male hormone testosterone is what makes men bulk up. Up to around age 12 to 14, boys and girls build the same amount of muscle. After that, once the testosterone kicks in, the guys are capable of building bigger muscles. Women don't tend to bulk up; they get toned.

Body type

There are three general body types: ectomorph, mesomorph, and endomorph. Ectomorphs are tall and thin; mesomorphs are muscular; and endomorphs tend to be short and plump. Most people have attributes from each body type. Bear in mind that it's harder for a tall, thin ectomorph to build muscle bulk, just as it is difficult for an endomorph to achieve unnatural slimness. Accept realistically what your body type is, and work with it. Genetics can't be changed; you're born a certain way, and you need to work with what you have.

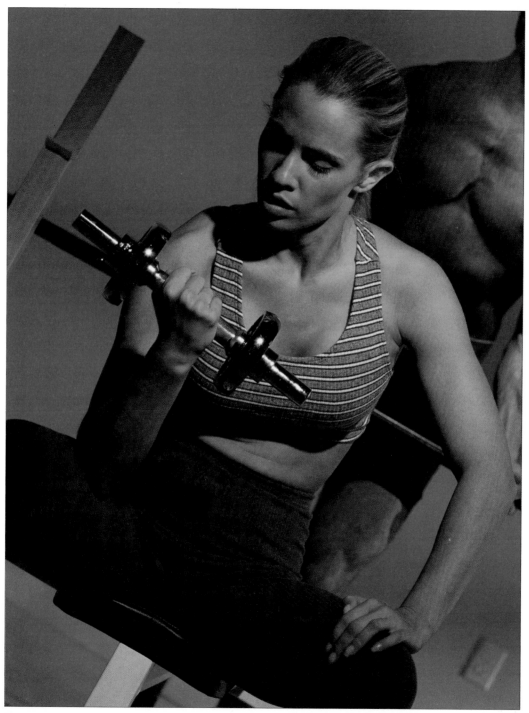

■ **Women who use weights** *tend to tone whereas men usually develop larger, heftier muscles. This is because men possess far greater quantities of the hormone testosterone, which causes them to bulk up.*

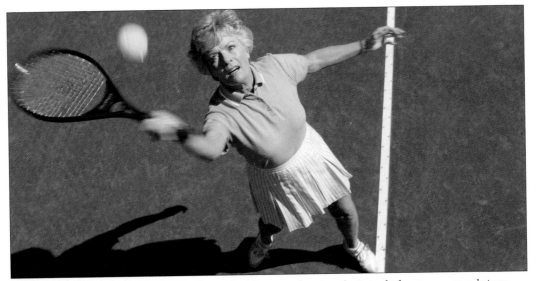

■ **The older you are**, *the longer it takes to build up muscle strength. But a little perseverance brings many benefits – not least of which is looking and feeling younger.*

Age

Another factor to consider is age. If you're over 35, don't expect to get toned as fast as you did when you were 17. Not that it can't be done eventually. But strength peaks in your 20s and declines after that. This doesn't mean you should hang up the barbells and plop down in the easy chair. It just means you should be aware and not get discouraged if you find it a little harder than it used to be to get toned.

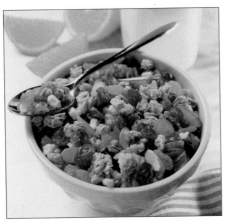

■ **A healthy diet** *is key to getting the most from any exercise regime. Eating balanced, low-fat meals will also help you lose weight.*

Diet

What you eat can certainly make a difference to how weight training affects you. If you're overweight, it's going to be harder to see those muscles underneath. Then again, if you're not eating enough, you won't have the energy to exercise hard. The best results come with combined exercise and a good diet. For more on nutrition, see Chapter 15.

If your primary exercise goal is to lose weight, concentrate on aerobic exercise and add the weight training in later.

Rest builds muscle

WEIGHT TRAINING IS SOMETHING to ease into. Even if you want to, you shouldn't lift weights every day. It's counterproductive. You need to give your muscles 48 hours between workouts – always, even as you progress. The skeletal muscles start to break down when exercised intensely more often than every other day. The day after intense exercise, bleeding and microscopic tearing can be seen in muscle fibres. That's why you feel sore after a good workout. That sounds bad but it's not, because the muscles are much stronger when they heal.

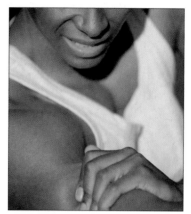

■ **Insufficient rest** *is a sure route to muscle strain.*

Resting allows the muscles to rebuild so they're bigger and stronger than before. Exercising intensely when the muscles ache can cause injury and decrease performance, but waiting for the muscles to stop aching before exercising intensely again strengthens the muscles. This is good news. No pain is, well, no pain. Period.

You should feel good after exercise. If you don't, you may have worked out too hard. Weight-training workouts should be hard enough so that the muscles are somewhat sore the next day, but fully recovered the day after that. If your muscles ache for days, you probably worked out too hard.

Sometimes the morning after I lift weights, I get up and say, "Hey! Nothing feels sore; I can't have worked out hard enough." But as the day progresses, "Ouch," suddenly that glass of water feels so heavy. The soreness doesn't hit me until a few hours later. Usually by the next day, the water glass isn't heavy any more, and my body feels okay again.

With all this in mind, you should plan to lift weights about two or three times a week, always giving yourself a day in between workouts. If you feel you really must, you can lift every day so long as you don't work on the same muscles. Some advanced weight lifters work on the upper body one day and the lower body the next without any trouble. Also, just because you shouldn't lift weights every day doesn't mean you can't get in some aerobics or stretching on the other days. Unlike lifting weights, you can stretch or do aerobic exercise every day without a problem.

Get results

YOU'RE ALL SET TO START TONING *and shaping up. So how*
much weight should you lift? Beginners to weight training should start with
light weights and high repetitions, gradually increasing
the weight. Find a weight you can lift 8 to 12 times, for
one or two **sets**. *If you can't lift it 8 times, then the*
weight is too heavy; you should try something lighter.
If 12 **reps** *are too easy, then you need to increase the*
weight. You can avoid too much soreness by beginning
with light weights and progressing gradually. Be patient
and ease into a programme.

> ### DEFINITION
>
> *A* **rep** *is short for repetition.*
> *It refers to one full range of*
> *motion. You do a certain*
> *number of reps for each* **set**.
> *For example, if you do three*
> *sets of ten reps, that means*
> *you lift ten times, rest, and*
> *repeat twice more.*

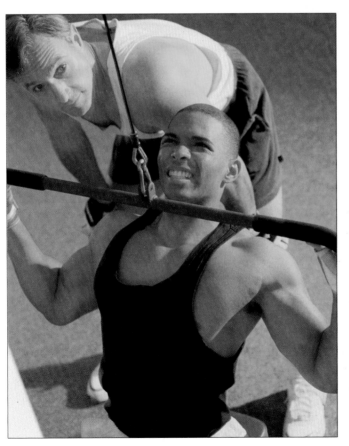

High reps (15–20 per set)
with low weight tones
muscles and improves
endurance. Low reps
(3–5 per set) of heavier
weight is good for strength
development. If you're just
starting a weight routine,
don't go with low reps of
high weights yet; start with
lower weight. Always rest for
about a minute between sets.
The rest period can vary
depending on your goals, but
a minute-long rest between
sets is perfect for beginners.

■ **A partner** *can help motivate*
you to push that little bit more, but
be sure to use good technique
throughout your reps – especially
when they are getting harder to do.

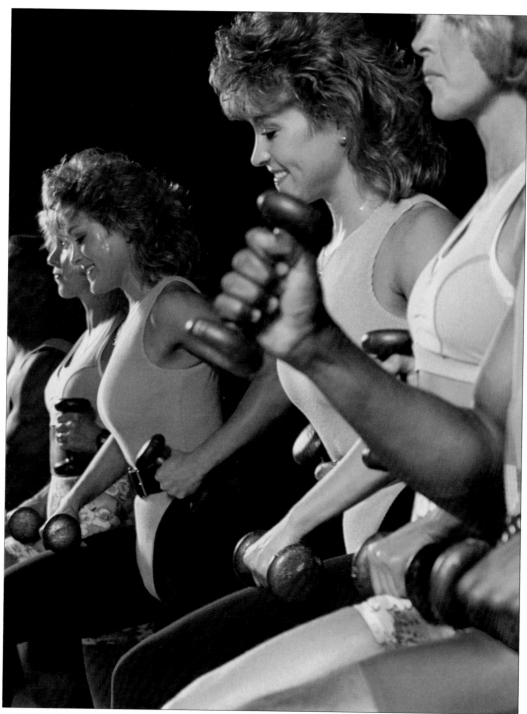

■ **Many body conditioning classes combine** *aerobic work with weight lifting. They're a good idea for beginners who want to get used to the feel of weights, and practise form in a motivational atmosphere.*

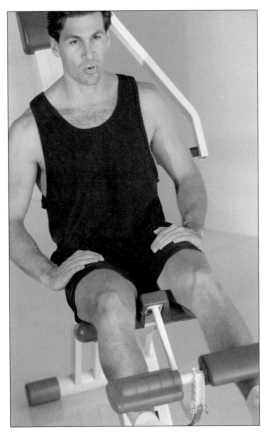

For most people, weight that can be lifted 8 to 12 times for three sets is appropriate for muscle growth and improved strength and endurance. For maximum strength and muscle development, sets should be done with weight heavy enough to cause muscle fatigue or the inability to do another rep. There is no ideal number of reps; as long as each set is the maximum number of reps you can do (within reason). If you can, schedule a few sessions with a personal trainer to help design the best workout for you.

Feel free to vary numbers of reps per set as well as the number of sets. There are no hard-and-fast rules. You might change your program whenever you get bored. If you stick to a program, your progress will probably start to plateau after 2 months. That will be a good time to change the program.

■ **Once you can comfortably lift** *a weight 8 to 12 times for three sets, you can increase the weight to a level that pushes you harder.*

Form is everything

THERE ARE A FEW BASIC GUIDELINES *for good form in weight lifting. We'll get more into the particular form of various exercises in Part Three, but in the meantime it's something to think about before you even start. It's important to have proper form to avoid injury. Form can make all the difference in your exercise program. Worst case is that bad form can cause injury; at the very least it can prevent you from getting the results you seek.*

- Never use momentum to swing the weight. Always use slow, controlled movements all the way up, holding, and all the way down. This way you're using the concentric and eccentric contraction
- Stay in control. Don't lift so much weight that you don't have control of the movement

- Keep your spine straight and relaxed
- Use a spotter – someone who's ready to grab the weight if you can't – when lifting free weights, especially heavy ones
- Breathe. Breathing can enhance your workout and actually make it easier to lift the weight. Exhale as you lift or exert force, contracting a muscle, and inhale as you lower, or release
- Completely flex and extend the joint you're working on, but don't lock the joint. If it's your arm, for example, don't over-extend your elbow
- Don't forget to warm up, stretch, and cool down

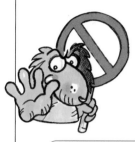

Never hold your breath when you lift weights.

A simple summary

✔ Muscles are a vital part of the human body. They determine the shape of our bodies and protect our bones, ligaments, and joints.

✔ Training with weights can do more than bulk up muscles. It can keep you toned, strengthen your bones, and make you stronger and more powerful.

✔ Every body is unique and will respond differently to weight training. If two people did the exact same weight training routine, chances are they'd get different results.

✔ Muscles are built after the workout. Always give yourself a day of rest between weight training sessions to give the muscles a chance to rebuild and get stronger.

✔ The best approach for beginners is to do high repetitions of lower weights. It's also the best way to get toned.

✔ Good form is important when lifting weights. Sloppy form can cause injury or no results.

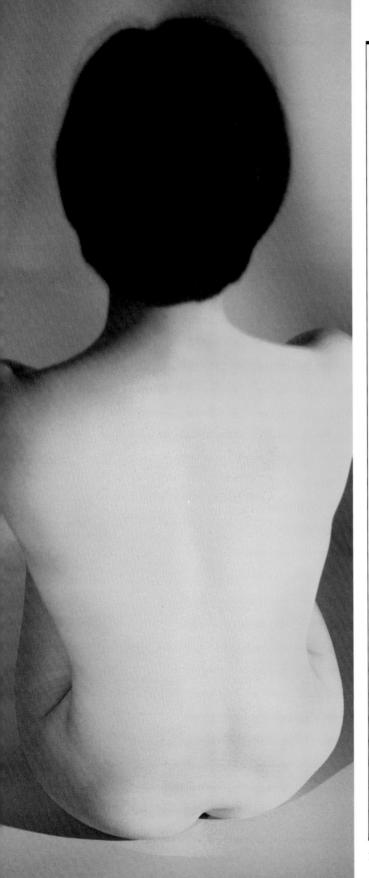

PART THREE

LEARN HOW TO GET THE BODY YOU ALWAYS WANTED

A FEW SIMPLE WORKOUTS

IN THIS SECTION, there's less talk and more action. Part Three is packed full of *exercises you can try at home* or at the *gym*. In addition, each selection includes a range to *suit every need* – including simple modifications to make your favourite exercise a little easier or to make it more challenging.

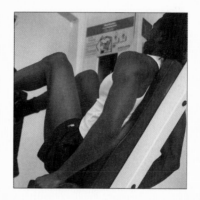

Take a look at *new ways to tone* your arms, back, and chest, to flatten that midsection, and to strengthen your legs. Revisit a few classic moves to give your entire body a workout. We'll do the push-ups and jumping jacks you may remember from P.E. lessons and a whole lot more. Tie on your shoes, find a spot in the garden, gym, or living room, and try these simple exercises that will get you toned in no time.

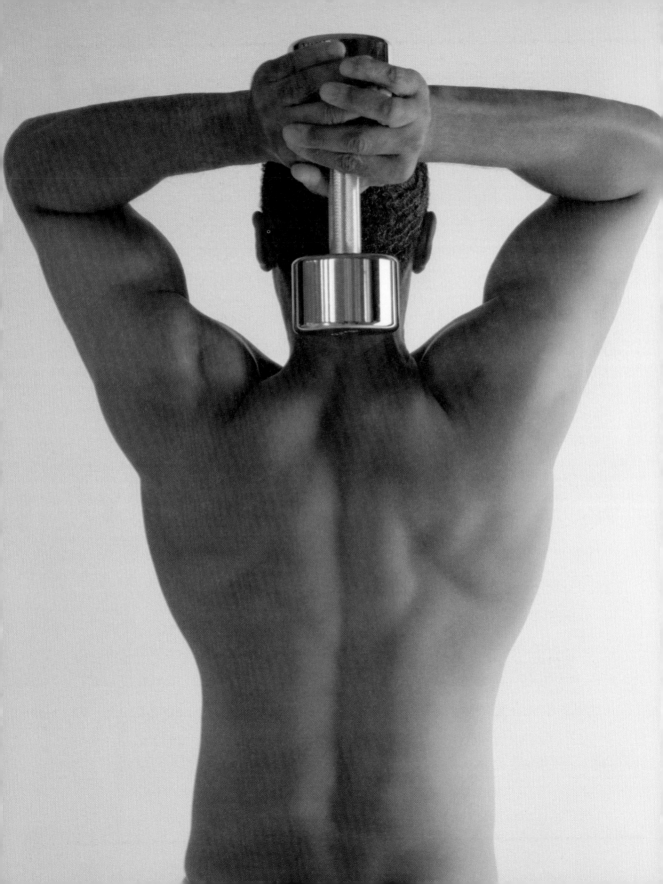

Chapter 11

Upper Body Workout

TONING AND STRENGTHENING your upper body has a lot of practical and aesthetic value. Strong arms, chest, and back can help you lift, pull, push – all moves you do every day. A toned upper body can keep you strong and healthy by strengthening your back to prevent injury. Learn how to do a total upper body workout with exercises you can try at home or at the gym.

In this chapter...

✔ Muscles in the upper body

✔ Why you need a strong upper body

✔ Up in arms

✔ Shoulders

✔ Chest

✔ Back

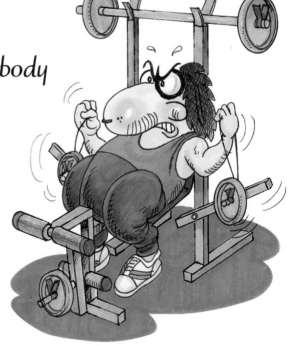

A DEFINED BACK CAN MAKE YOUR WAIST LOOK SMALLER

Muscles in the upper body

AS WE LEARNED IN THE LAST CHAPTER, *there are over 450 muscles in the human body. Here we'll concern ourselves with the muscles in the arm, shoulder, chest, and back.*

Let's look at some of the muscles we're going to tone:

a **Pectoral:** these chest muscles flex and rotate the arm, move the shoulders and are used in pushing and pulling

b **Latissimus dorsi:** the largest muscle in the back, this runs diagonally across the lower back. It extends and rotates the arm, draws the shoulder down and back, and helps in climbing

c **Trapezius:** this is the large muscle that runs along the upper back and neck area. It raises, turns, and lowers the shoulders and turns the face to the same or opposite side

d **Biceps:** so-named because they have two parts, these muscles run along the front of the arm, flexing the arm and forearm and turning the palm upwards

e **Triceps:** thus named because there are three parts, these extend the arm and forearm and can move the arm in towards the body

f **Deltoids:** the shoulder is made up of three parts: the front, middle, and rear deltoids. These muscles are often referred to as one unit. The deltoids are important for flexing and rotating the arm inwards and extending and moving the arm away from the body

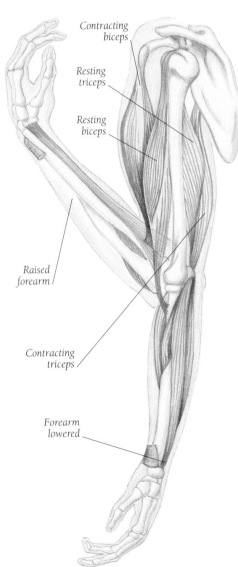

Contracting biceps

Resting triceps

Resting biceps

Raised forearm

Contracting triceps

Forearm lowered

■ **The biceps and triceps muscles** *are arranged so that as one contracts, the other relaxes to give a smooth, controlled movement.*

Why you need a strong upper body

OF COURSE, WE DON'T WANT *you toning up unevenly, so work in your upper body exercises with those for the lower body and abs. A strong upper body can help you with your daily activities such as lifting and carrying babies or bags of shopping, pushing open a stuck door, or winning an all-important arm wrestling contest.*

The upper body is also the part that other people see the most. Not that it matters of course, since we're doing this for ourselves, but still – it's nice to look toned and healthy.

Arms, in particular, respond to strength training very quickly. You could possibly see results in as little as 2 weeks. Biceps tone up fast, and show. Also, working the triceps is good for toning up that back-of-the-arm flab that can make you want to wear long sleeves all summer.

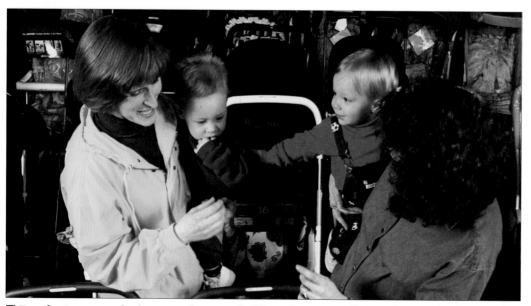

■ **Developing upper body strength** *can make life much easier in all sorts of practical ways. Carrying and lifting babies and toddlers, for example, is less tiring when your muscles are in good shape.*

Up in arms

LET'S START WITH THE ARMS then. First we'll go through a few exercises you can do without weights. Then we'll try a few with small hand weights.

Push-ups

Muscles worked: chest and arms (triceps, pectoral muscles, and latissimus dorsi).

Push-ups are a tried-and-true way to shape up.

Keep a straight line from your head to your hips; don't arch or sway your back.

Incline push-ups

This is a good way to start because incline push-ups aren't quite as difficult to do as push-ups on the floor lifting all your body weight. These can help you get the hang of a push-up. Incline push-ups can be done using a tree, wall, chair, or any other sturdy object that provides an incline for you to push against.

1. Face the wall, standing about 1 metre (3 ft) in front of it with your feet shoulder-width apart

2. Reach out and put your hands on the wall. Keeping your spine straight and your head and neck in a straight line, bend your arms and inhale as you slowly lower your body to the wall (or tree, etc.). Don't let your head bend forwards or backwards, and try to get as close as possible to the wall

3. Hold the position for 2–3 seconds; then exhale and slowly push away. Concentrate on contracting your pectoral and triceps muscles

INCLINE PUSH-UP

Modified push-ups

Once you've mastered the incline push-up, try the modified push-up. These push-ups are done with your body weight balanced on your hands and the area just above your knee joint. Don't rest your weight directly on your kneecap (patella) as this could damage your knee.

1 Get down on your hands and knees. Slide your knees back so that they're at slightly more than a 90-degree angle to ensure that you're resting on the spot above your kneecap. Your feet can be in the air or on the floor

2 Bend your arms and inhale as you slowly lower your chest to within 7.5 cm (3 in) of the floor

3 Exhale as you straighten your arms and slowly return to the starting position. Remember to lower and lift your body as a single unit; don't let it bend or sag

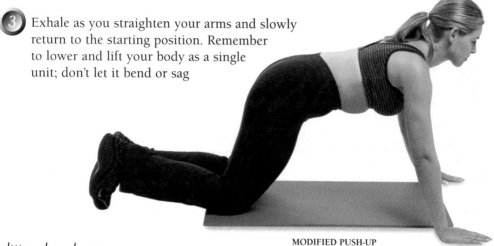

MODIFIED PUSH-UP

Traditional push-ups

When you think of a push-up, this is the one you're probably thinking of. Traditional push-ups are also called military push-ups.

1 Lie face down on the floor. Put your hands under your shoulders, and raise your body onto your toes and hands. Keep your abdominal muscles contracted and your spine in a neutral position (not arched or swayed), and keep your body stabilized throughout the full range of motion during this exercise

2 Inhale and bend your elbows as you slowly lower your body to within 7.5 cm (3 in) of the floor. Exhale as you push back up to the starting position

3 If you feel any pain or strain in your lower back, stop and go back to the modified push-ups until you build up enough strength to do this variation. Take your time and develop proper form and strength. You can start building endurance by alternating sets of military push-ups and modified ones

TIPS FOR PUSH-UPS

To help you get maximum benefit from all push-up exercises, here are some guidelines:

1 Your palms should be on the floor a little wider than shoulder-width apart

2 Try to do two sets of 12 reps. If that's too hard, start slowly and work your way up. Once you've mastered two sets of 12 reps, increase the reps or sets, or move on to the next push-up variation

Trivia...

Do not try this at home. In 1980, Minoru Yoshida of Japan broke the Guinness world record for non stop push-ups. He did 10,507 traditional push-ups without stopping!

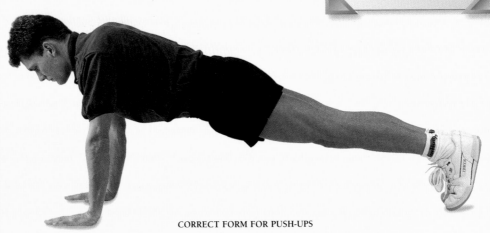

CORRECT FORM FOR PUSH-UPS

3 Do a quick stretch between sets. With your hands and knees on the floor, extend your arms out in front and bring your hips back to your heels. Rest your forehead on the floor and breathe. This is also called the "child's pose" in yoga

Where you place your hands while doing push-ups affects the muscles you build. If you do push-ups with your arms further than shoulder-width apart, you work your outer chest muscles more. If your hands are closer together, the triceps and inner chest muscles get a better workout. Vary your hand position to tighten the different parts of the chest.

Triceps dips

Muscles worked: triceps.

This is a difficult upper body exercise, but a great way to tone the triceps so you can wave to someone while wearing short sleeves and not worry about what's shaking underneath your arm.

For this you need a stable chair or a ledge that's about 60 cms (2 ft) off the ground. If you're using a chair, you might want to prop it up against the wall so it doesn't slide out behind you.

1. Reach behind you and hold on to the edge of the chair (or ledge) with both hands (palms down, fingers forward); then slide your rear forward and off the seat

STEP 1

2. Bending at the elbow, lower your body toward the ground and then raise it back up. Push with your arms. To make it easier, bring your legs in; to make it more challenging, extend legs out far in front

3. Try two sets of 12 reps

Chin-ups

Muscles worked: arms and back (latissimus dorsi, trapezius, biceps, triceps, and deltoids).

Chin-ups are an efficient and quick way to tone many of the muscles in your arms, chest, and back. All you need is a bar – a chin-up bar at home, an apparatus at the gym, or just hang on the monkey bars at the playground. For more information about chin-up bars, see Chapter 5.

1. Grab the bar at about shoulder width, with your palms facing you. Begin from a hanging position with your elbows fully extended

2. Keeping your chest up and shoulder blades pulled back, pull your body up to the bar until your chin is just above the bar. Pause briefly at the top before slowly returning to the starting position with your elbows extended

3. Instead of counting on this one, do as many as you can

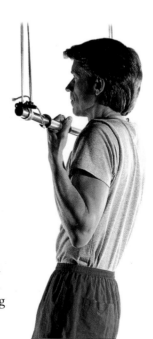

STEP 2

Chin-ups are really difficult. If you can't do the chin-up on the previous page, try this modified version. If you have a helpful friend, have your friend spot you by holding your feet, ankles, or legs to take some of the weight. The spotter may have to take a great deal of weight depending on how difficult the movement is for the lifter. Try it a few times like this until you can do it on your own. Find a partner, and you can take turns helping each other on this one.

Now it's time to pick up some weights

For the next few exercises, you need a couple of hand weights. For beginners, women should try 1.3–2.2 kg (3–5 lb) weights, and men should try 3.5–6 kg (8–15 lb) weights. As we discussed in Chapter 10, if you can't lift the weight eight times, it's too heavy; you should try something a bit lighter. If you can lift it 12 times easily, try a higher weight.

Biceps curls

Muscles worked: biceps.

The biceps curl is one of my favourites because the basic movement is simple, but the biceps show the effort quickly. This means you can soon impress your friends with your lovely new biceps.

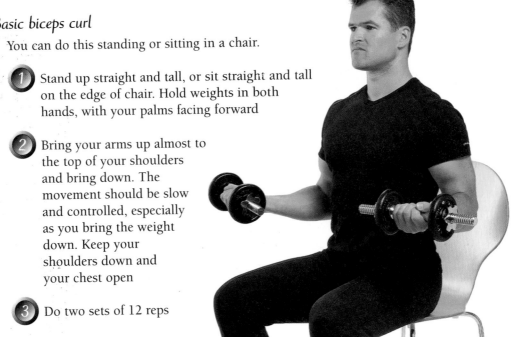

Basic biceps curl

You can do this standing or sitting in a chair.

1. Stand up straight and tall, or sit straight and tall on the edge of chair. Hold weights in both hands, with your palms facing forward

2. Bring your arms up almost to the top of your shoulders and bring down. The movement should be slow and controlled, especially as you bring the weight down. Keep your shoulders down and your chest open

3. Do two sets of 12 reps

STEP 2

ADVANCED CURLS: "21s"

This advanced move breaks the basic biceps curl down into three parts. If you want to concentrate on the arm movement, you can also sit in a chair for this one.

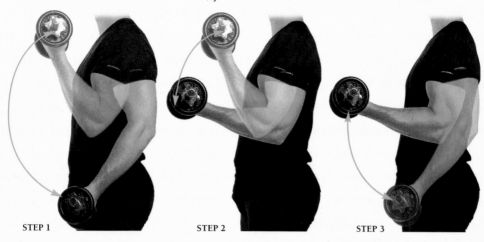

STEP 1　　　　　STEP 2　　　　　STEP 3

1 Hold the weight in one hand, down by your side. First, do seven full biceps curls – all the way up and all the way down

2 Next, start from the midpoint (forearm parallel to floor) and bring it all the way up and back down to the midpoint for seven reps

3 Without stopping, lower your arm to the starting point again and lift from the bottom to the midpoint seven times

4 Switch the weight to the other hand and repeat. You should really feel this one

5 You are welcome to do two sets, but one round should be plenty

Never sacrifice quantity for quality. If the weight is so heavy that you're swaying and leaning and feel out of control, try a lighter weight. It's better to do three reps with good form than ten reps with bad form.

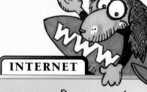

INTERNET

www.fitpro.com/
news/exerwat/exerwat
0898.html

Log on here to read everything you ever wanted to know about the biceps and more.

One-arm triceps extension

Muscles worked: triceps.

1 Stand with your feet parallel and shoulder-width apart. Hold the weight in one hand. Bend that arm, and place the other hand behind your elbow (in front of your chest)

2 Lift your elbow up towards the ceiling while keeping your shoulder down. The weight should be behind your ear. Extend and straighten your arm up – extend the weight up as high as possible to stretch your triceps

3 Slowly bend the arm back to starting position. Keep the opposite hand on the arm that's doing the lifting to keep it steady. The upper arm should be still during the movement

4 Do two to three sets of 12 reps with each arm

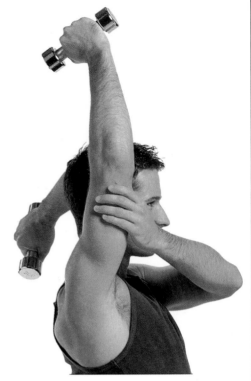

ONE-ARM TRICEPS EXTENSION

Shoulders

SOME OF THE ABOVE EXERCISES *work the shoulders as well as the lower part of the arm, but to get your arms into really top condition, it's important to have a few dedicated shoulder exercises in your routine. Here are a couple of moves that focus on the shoulder. These can help you develop a fully toned and strengthened arm.*

Shoulder raises

Muscles worked: deltoids.

This exercise works the front, middle, and rear deltoids. Toned deltoids can give you a nice shoulder cap, which is a smooth rounded shoulder that comes from training the muscles that run from the top to the centre of your upper arm.

1. Start in a standing position, with your feet shoulder-width apart, abs in, chest out

2. Pinch your shoulder blades together. Hold a weight in each hand, with both hands down by your sides and palms in. With your elbows slightly bent, lift arms out to the side and away from your body

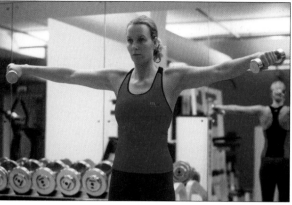

STEP 2

When doing shoulder raises, never let your arms go higher than shoulder height.

3. Slowly bring your arms back down to your sides. Then, from the same starting position, lift arms out in front, once again not going higher than shoulder height

4. Do 12 reps of six to the side and six to the front; then repeat for a total of two sets

Overhead press

Muscles worked: mainly shoulders (deltoids); also back (latissimus dorsi) and biceps

1. From a standing position, feet shoulder-width apart, hold both your weights with your arms down by your sides and palms facing in

2. Bend your elbows and bring your arms up so that your arms are parallel to the floor. The weights should be just in front of your temples. Then lift both arms straight up over your head. You should be able to see your elbows in your peripheral vision, otherwise your arms are back too far

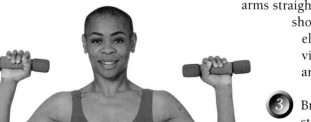

OVERHEAD PRESS

3. Bring each arm back down to starting position (with your upper arm parallel to the floor), and repeat. Keep your abs in tight, and don't lean back

185

Chest

TONING THE CHEST IS GOOD, *at least partly because it's what you see in the mirror. Working this area can give men a sculpted chest. Although breasts are made up of fat tissue, women can build the muscle underneath to create a firmer and sometimes larger chest.*

Chest press

Muscles worked: chest (pectoral muscles).

1. Lie on the floor with a pillow under your shoulders and head, and place a towel behind your neck for more support

2. Bend your knees, and press your feet and back firmly into the floor. Abdominals should be pulled in tight. Place your hands at chest level, with your palms facing your knees

3. Holding a weight in each hand, raise your arms overhead, palms still facing your knees. Using slow, controlled movements, lower your hands to your chest. Don't go past the shoulders with your elbows. Raise your arms back above you. Don't lock your elbows

4. Work up to two sets of 12 reps

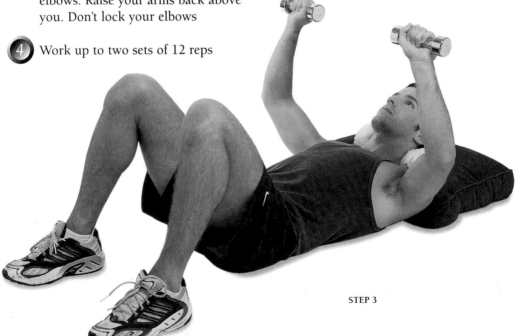

STEP 3

Fly

Muscles worked: chest (pectoral muscles).

1 Start in a lying position, as for the chest press. Holding a weight in each hand, raise arms overhead, and turn the palms inward so that they face each other

2 Lower your arms straight out to the sides, maintaining a slight bend in the elbows throughout the exercise. Exhale as you squeeze up

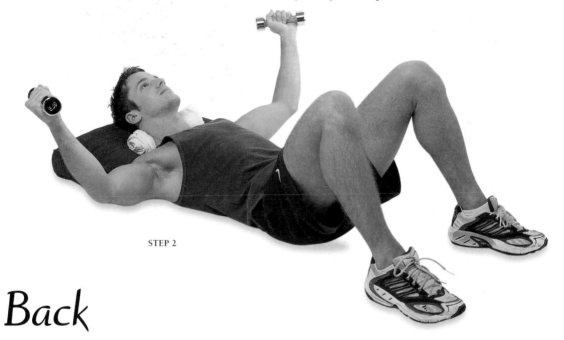

STEP 2

Back

STRENGTHENING YOUR BACK *is one of the best things you can do to improve your posture and alleviate back pain. Toning up your back reduces your chances of injury from everyday lifting and activities.*

If you've had back trouble in the past, be very careful when doing back exercises. A strong back can prevent problems later, but make sure to get that strong back safely.

Strengthening your upper back and the back of your shoulders is important in helping maintain good posture. Weak upper back muscles cause your shoulders to slump forward and can eventually result in neck problems. Also, a defined back can give you the appearance of having a smaller waist.

Bentover flies

Muscles worked: shoulder and back (the rear deltoid and the trapezius).

Start this one with lighter weight because this is a challenging lift.

1 Sit on the edge of a chair, with your ankles directly underneath your knees. Arms should be down by your sides, with a weight in each hand

2 Pull your shoulders down so they're not up by your ears. Hingeing at the hip, bend over so that your chest is over your thighs. Let your abs support you; don't lean on your legs. Your forehead faces the floor. Bring your shoulder blades together in the back

3 Bring your arms out to the sides, away from your body. Slowly bring them back down to the edge of your heels

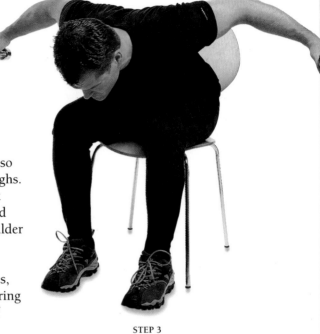

STEP 3

4 Do two sets of 12 reps. Remember that these are a little harder, so try it first with lighter weight and build up

One-arm row

Muscles worked: mostly the latissimus dorsi; also back of the shoulder (rear deltoid) and the biceps.

1 Place your left knee on a bench or chair with your left hip aligned directly over it. The knee of the right leg should be at about the same height and slightly bent. Place your left hand on the front edge of the bench. Let your fingers curl over the edge of the bench rather than placing it flat on the bench. (This position helps protect your wrist from discomfort.) Your upper body should be parallel to the floor. The dumbbell should be on the floor near your right foot

2 Lower your body to pick up the weight and return to this start position with your arm hanging straight down

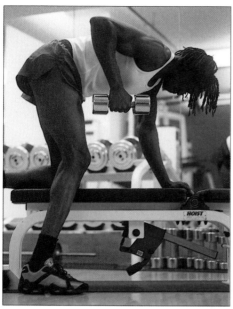

STEP 4

3 Hold the dumbbell without tilting it and keep your wrist straight. Rotate your shoulder so that your elbow is pointing away from your side. Try to pinch your shoulder blades together, and keep this position throughout the exercise

4 Bend your elbow and pull the weight up until your upper arm is parallel to the floor or higher and your elbow forms a right angle. Keep your abs pulled in tight. This will help support your lower back. Also, keep your chest square to the floor. Pause and return the weight to the starting position

5 Do two sets of 12 reps; then change sides and repeat

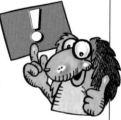

If your arms are getting tired, you aren't using your back muscles enough.

A simple summary

✓ There are many muscles in the upper body alone.

✓ Toning the muscles in the upper body can not only help us look and feel great but can help us with daily tasks like lifting, pulling, and pushing.

✓ Push-ups, triceps dips, biceps curls, and triceps extensions can shape up your arms in no time.

✓ There are many exercises to create a rounded shoulder, such as shoulder raises and the overhead press.

✓ The chest gets shapely with push-ups, chest presses, and flies.

✓ Develop a strong back with bentover flies and one-arm rows.

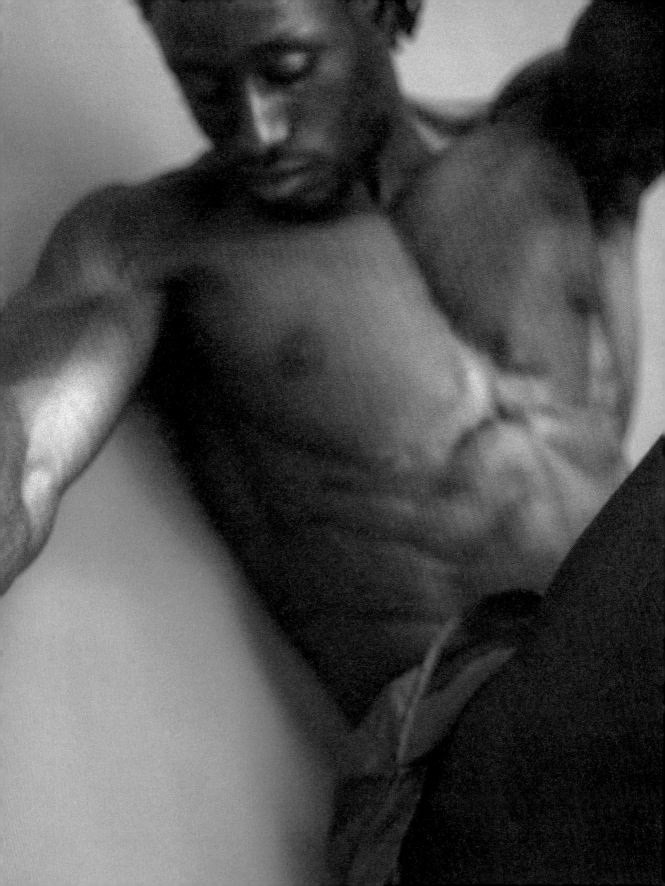

Chapter 12

Get a Flat Stomach

HAVING A TONED AND FLAT MIDSECTION LOOKS GREAT and increases overall strength and balance. Firming up abdominal muscles provides extra support to the back to prevent or alleviate back pain. Toned abs also help performance in everything from daily tasks to sports. We'll take a look at the muscles that make up the abdomen, learn what they do, and check out exercises designed to work every part of the abdominal area.

In this chapter...

✓ Muscles in the torso

✓ Why you need strong abdominal muscles

✓ Tips on abdominal exercises

✓ Abdominal workouts

✓ Obliques

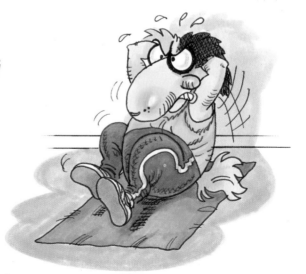

STRONG ABDOMINAL MUSCLES IMPROVE BALANCE AND POSTURE AND HELP PROTECT THE SPINE

Muscles in the torso

THE ABDOMINAL MUSCLES ("abs") are the large group of muscles in front of the abdomen. This group of muscles assists regular breathing movement and supports the muscles of the spine while lifting. It also keeps the abdominal organs, such as the intestines, in place.

Let's take a look at some of the muscles we're going to tone:

(a) **Rectus abdominis:** this one runs down the middle, the entire length of the abdominal area. This muscle stabilizes the trunk and pulls the sternum (breastbone) toward the hips and the hips toward the sternum. In addition, it tilts the pelvis, in turn affecting the curvature of the spine

The rectus abdominis is the most superficial abdominal muscle, the one that's closest to the surface. This is the one you can see when you develop your ab muscles. It's the one that gives you the "six pack" or "washboard stomach" look.

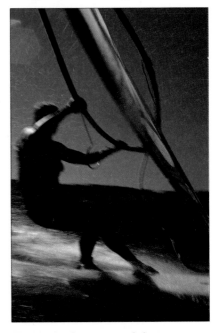

■ **Toning the rectus abdominis** *can enhance performance in sports in which you have to lift, such as windsurfing, and those in which you run and jump, such as track events or wrestling.*

(b) **Transversus abdominis:** this is the deepest abdominal muscle. It runs horizontally across the abdominal wall and along the midsection underneath the external and internal obliques (see below). The transversus abdominis pulls the abdominal wall inward and forces the breath out. Toning this large muscle can enhance activities that need short bursts of power such as karate, kickboxing, or football

(c) **External oblique:** this muscle runs along your side, diagonally to the rectus abdominis. It forms a V across the front of the abdominal area, extending diagonally down from the lower ribs to the pubic bone, and helps twist the trunk. You use the left external oblique when twisting to the right and activate the right external oblique when you twist to the left. Strengthening this area can help improve your performance in any activity in which you have to rotate your trunk, such as tennis, golf, or baseball

(d) **Internal oblique:** this muscle lies under the external oblique and runs in a diagonally opposed direction. The internal oblique helps twist the trunk in the direction of the side it is on. The left internal oblique helps the torso twist to the left and helps the right external oblique in this movement. The right internal oblique helps twist the torso to the right and helps the left external oblique. Strengthening this area can also help with activities in which you have to rotate your trunk, especially football, paddling (canoe, kayak), or skiing

Why you need strong abdominal muscles

NOT ONLY DO FIRM, STRONG ABS look attractive, they're important for overall strength. They're the centre of your body, and they're part of every movement. They assist in the regular breathing movement and support the muscles of the spine while lifting and keeping the abdominal organs in place. They're the core of your strength and power.

Strong abdominal muscles can alleviate back pain and increase your general fitness. Toned abs play an important role in stabilizing the spine and pelvis. Contracting the ab muscles increases pressure within the abdomen, which then pushes against the back and helps the back stabilize itself. This is helpful in all sorts of everyday activities, from lifting objects to playing sports.

As with all strength-training exercises, you'll need to get into a healthy weight range before you begin to see a lot of muscle definition.

If you want results fast, combine abdominal exercises with a sensible low-fat diet.

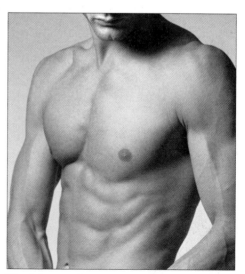

■ **Abdominal exercises** *will tone your mid-section but you need to be in a healthy weight range in order to really see muscle definition – otherwise the fat will hide your progress.*

Tips on abdominal exercises

THE MAIN MOVEMENT *of the abdominal muscles is to shorten the distance between the sternum (breastbone) and the pelvis. To work the abs, do exercises that move your sternum towards your pelvis or your pelvis towards your sternum. Keep this in mind as you do the exercises. The point is to prevent lifting from the neck or using other muscles.*

It helps to visualize the correct movements as you do them; so, when you're working your abdominal muscles, concentrate on using them to shorten the distance between your sternum and pelvis. Imagine your abs doing this as you exercise.

Crunches vs. sit-ups

Crunches are, loosely, a type of sit-up. Although there are variations, a classic sit-up is the motion in which you're on your back and you pull your upper body all the way up and all the way back down for one sit-up.

Few fitness experts still promote this kind of sit-up because it can hurt your back, especially if your legs are straight. I recently had to perform this kind of sit-up (bent knee, not straight) for a fitness test, so they are still around. (I was sore for days!) The words "sit-ups" and "crunches" are often thrown around as meaning the same thing, but basically, crunches are smaller, more subtle movements that isolate an area.

> ## Trivia...
> *Unanchored (feet not tucked under anything or held down), straight-legged sit-ups were popular until sports scientists concluded that the hip flexors were too involved and the abs weren't doing enough work. They also decided that there was a chance of injuring the lower back with this type of sit-up. Bending the knees reduces the chance of hurting the lower back.*

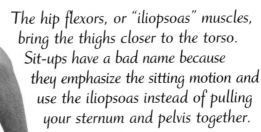

The hip flexors, or "iliopsoas" muscles, bring the thighs closer to the torso. Sit-ups have a bad name because they emphasize the sitting motion and use the iliopsoas instead of pulling your sternum and pelvis together.

■ **Crunches** *(shown here) are safer and more effective than traditional sit-ups because they isolate the abs area and don't strain the back.*

GENERAL EXERCISE TIPS

Here are some general tips for ab exercises to keep you safe and get you strong:

1. Your lower back should be slightly rounded, not arched. Maintain a neutral spine or press it slightly down into the mat. Don't arch your back when doing ab exercises. Your lower back will probably round a bit as you do the ab exercises

2. Never pull with your neck; always move from the midsection. If your hands are behind your head, keep them there lightly and don't pull your head up with your hands

3. Use a mat or towel on a carpet to protect your lower back from a hard floor

4. If you feel any sharp pain, stop what you're doing. A little discomfort as you exert yourself is okay, but sharp or sudden pain is never okay when exercising

Keep the tension in your abdominal area during the entire exercise.

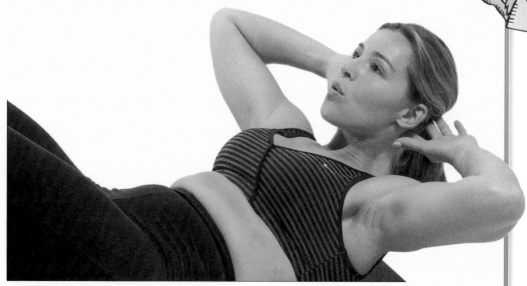

■ **Don't hold your breath** *when doing ab exercises. Exhale on the exertion and inhale on the release. If that's too much to think about at first, just breathe naturally.*

Abdominal workouts

HERE IS A LIST OF EXERCISES *designed to work your entire abdominal region. You're bound to have heard of some of these, but you'll find additional variations to try. Try them all and find which ones work best for you. Also, mix it up. Doing the exact same ab routine every day is not only boring; it can even make it harder to progress. I recommend working up to 20 reps of each of these, but you can do more if you feel up to it. Do as many as you can. With these exercises it's okay to feel the burn.*

All the exercises that follow have been designed to hit each part of the abdominal section without causing pain to the lower back.

If you find any movement uncomfortable, move on to the next one for now. Also, don't push yourself to a more difficult exercise until you are ready.

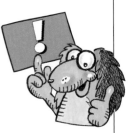

Pelvic tilt

This is a good move to start with. The exercise is a subtle movement that will help get your back into the correct position for doing abdominal exercises.

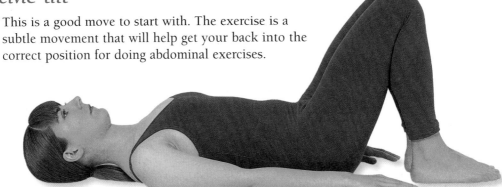

PELVIC TILT

1. Begin by lying on your back on a mat (or towel) with your knees bent

2. Tighten your stomach and flatten your back into the floor. Your feet should remain flat on the floor while you hold this position for 6 seconds. Really press your lower back into the floor

3. Slowly release and return to the original position

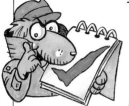

The pelvic tilt is a good beginning exercise as it helps you get a feel for pressing your back into the mat, which is what you'll want to do when executing these ab exercises.

Any ab exercise you do will affect your entire midsection because the abdominal muscles work together. But different exercises stress the upper, lower, and side. The exercises listed below go from working the upper abs, to the lower abs, to the sides to give the entire abdominal area a full tune-up. Basically, the three types of ab exercises are those that require lifting from the chest, like crunches, those that require lifting from the pelvis, such as leg raises, and rotating exercises like the torso twists.

Crunches

The **crunch** has replaced the sit-up as the most popular abdominal exercise. This movement mostly works the upper abdomen. There are many variations. Here are some of my favourites:

> **DEFINITION**
>
> *With a **crunch**, you lift your upper body – head, shoulders, and upper back – but your lower back stays on the floor.*

Basic crunch

1 Lie on your back on a mat with knees bent, feet hip-width apart and flat on the floor at a comfortable distance from your rear. (You may need to experiment to find a good spot for your feet.) Cross your arms in front of you with hands on opposite shoulders

2 Tighten your stomach and lift your head, neck, and chest up as one unit. Lift your shoulder blades off the floor. Concentrate on pulling your chest down towards your hips. Keep your glutes relaxed and a neutral spine position. Exhale as you lift up and hold for a count of two

3 Slowly lower down to the floor while inhaling

4 Work up to one set of 20

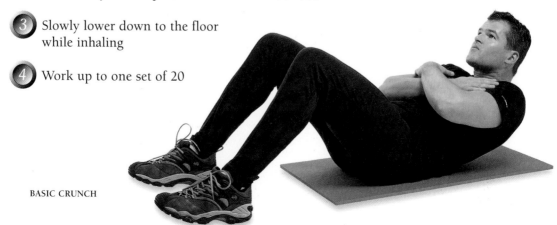

BASIC CRUNCH

Crunch variations

Once you get comfortable with the basic crunch, try the following variations. Changing your arm position can make a difference in the intensity of the move.

Variation 1: another way to do a crunch is the same as above, but put your hands behind your head with your elbows out.

Don't pull your head up with your hands. If you're not sure whether or not you're doing this, move your hands away from your head every so often, and see if your head stays in the same position.

Variation 2: if you want a little more challenge, hold your arms straight out in front of you, and hold them out as you lift and lower.

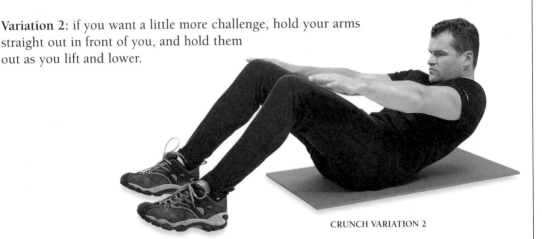

CRUNCH VARIATION 2

Variation 3: from the same position as the basic crunch, put your feet up on a chair or ledge so your calves are parallel to the floor. Bring your upper body up just as you would with a basic crunch.

CRUNCH VARIATION 3

Reverse crunch

The next three movements – reverse crunch, lying leg raise, and hanging knee raise – work the entire midsection, but focus on the lower abdomen. With these moves, you're lifting from your lower body instead of from your upper body.

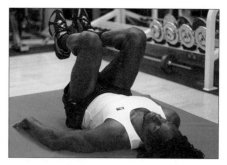

REVERSE CRUNCH

1. Lie on your back on a mat with your back flat against the floor and arms down by your sides

2. Raise your legs in the air with hips and knees both bent to 90 degrees. (Shins should be parallel to the floor)

3. Raise your rear and pull hips off the floor while contracting abdominals in a slow motion. Hold for 2 seconds, then lower. Don't just raise your legs; concentrate on raising your pelvis towards your stomach. This is a small concentrated movement. Go slowly and stay in control; don't let momentum do the work for you. Make sure you're forcing your abs to do the work

4. Work up to 20 reps

Lying leg raise

1. Lie on your back with your hands, palms down, under your buttocks

2. Raise your legs about 30 cm (12 in) off the floor and hold them there

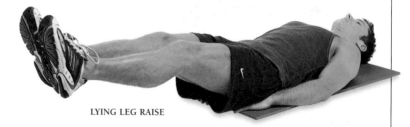

LYING LEG RAISE

3. Now, trying to use just your lower abs, raise your legs by another 15 cm (6 in). Do this by tilting your pelvis instead of lifting your legs with your hips. Hold at the top for a few seconds, then lower back down. Make sure your knees are slightly bent and not locked

4. Try to do 20 reps

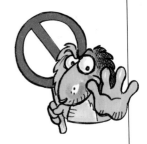

Be very careful not to arch your back when doing the lying leg raise. If your legs are heavy, or if you find that your lower back is being pulled into an exaggerated arch, or if it's painful at all, bend your knees slightly and try to keep a flat back – or just miss out the leg raise altogether.

Hanging knee raise

This is an advanced move for which you need a chin-up bar or something you can hang from.

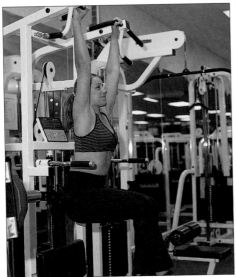

HANGING KNEE RAISE

1. Reach up and grab the bar with your hands a little further than shoulder-width apart

2. Cross your ankles and bring your knees up to your chest (or as close as you can get), pausing briefly at the top, and then slowly lower your legs back to the starting position by relaxing your abs. Your pelvis should rock slightly forward. Don't lower your legs all the way

3. Repeat the movement using just your abs to raise your knees. Make sure that you don't start swinging. Again, you want your abs to do the work, not momentum

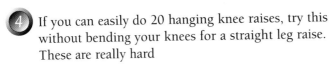

Don't move your legs too far when doing hanging knee raises. Make sure your pelvis moves, your lower back stays neutral or slightly rounded, not arched, and that your abs are doing the work, not your hips.

4. If you can easily do 20 hanging knee raises, try this without bending your knees for a straight leg raise. These are really hard

INTERNET

www.t-mag.com/
html/body_123abs.html

www.fitnesslink.com/
women/moreabs.shtml

For specialized information on abs – exercises, tips, training – men should go to the first site listed above, and women should check out the second site.

Obliques

THE FOLLOWING EXERCISES *work
the external and internal obliques, which are
the muscles that you use when you twist or
rotate your torso from side to side. For these,
in addition to thinking about bringing your
sternum and pelvis together, imagine your sides
working to rotate your torso. Toning this area
can help provide support for the lower back.*

Standing torso twist

Here is a good move for beginners. For this one,
forget about bringing your sternum and pelvis
together and just think about using your obliques
to twist. Strengthen your obliques with this twisting
movement of your trunk.

1. Stand with your feet shoulder-width apart,
   with your hands behind your head and
   elbows straight out to the side

2. Rotate your torso 90 degrees to the left, so
   that you're facing the left side with your
   upper body, but your feet and legs still face
   forward. Think about leading with your
   shoulder. Hold for a beat, tighten the abs,
   then return to the starting position

3. Repeat on the same side 15–20 times; then do
   the same thing on the right side. Don't rush
   through. Make sure you hold the twist position
   for a second before you return to centre

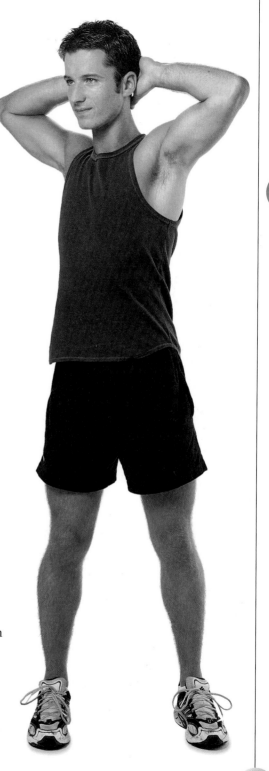

■ **The standing torso twist** *and other exercises that work the
external and internal obliques can help get rid of "love handles".*

201

Torso twist

This movement starts off like a bent-knee sit-up or crunch except that instead of bringing your upper torso straight up, you turn or twist your torso to the side during each repetition.

1 Start out as if you were going to do a crunch, that is lie back on a mat (or towel), knees bent and feet hip-width part. Place hands behind your head with your elbows out to the sides

2 Pull up as if you were doing a crunch, but while lifted rotate one shoulder towards the opposite knee. Don't pull with your elbow or twist just your neck; rotate your upper body. Think about bringing your armpit to the opposite knee

3 Come back down and repeat on the other side

To make the torso twist still more challenging and to work the obliques even more, twist to both sides at the top of the lift. Lift up, rotate left, rotate right, and down.

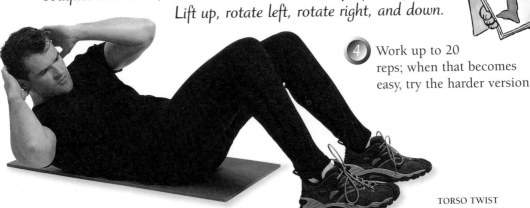

4 Work up to 20 reps; when that becomes easy, try the harder version

TORSO TWIST

Bicycles

Here's a move that is a little more challenging, but it's fun and very effective.

1 Lie on your back on a mat with both knees bent at a 90-degree angle (shins parallel to the floor). Place your hands behind your head with your elbows pointed out. Keep your spine neutral (don't arch it) and abs tight

2 Extend right leg out while pulling left knee in toward your chest. Simultaneously raise your shoulders and twist your trunk so your right shoulder and elbow approach your left knee. Hold for 1 second; then repeat with opposite side

3 Alternate for 20 reps (two twists equals one rep)

Half sit-up with twist

1 Lie on your back with your feet hip-width apart and flat on the ground. You can hook them under something or have someone hold your feet down, or just try to keep your feet on the floor. Cross your arms in front of you, with your left hand on your right shoulder and right hand on left shoulder

2 Rise up and bring your left elbow to your right knee, go back down halfway, and rise back up and bring your right elbow to your left knee

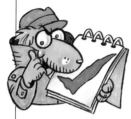

The half sit-up with twist is my favourite. I remember it from P.E. lessons at school. For this one, I try hook my toes under something and do a quick 50 in the morning before I get dressed. These days, the powers that be say not to hold your feet down – but it's much harder (and thus, more beneficial) that way.

A simple summary

✔ The abdomen is made up of a complex network of muscles including the rectus abdominis, transversus abdominis, external oblique, and internal oblique.

✔ Strong abs can enhance your performance in sports, increase your strength and balance for everyday activities, and can, quite frankly, make you look very fit.

✔ When doing ab exercises, it's important not to arch your back, hold your breath, or pull with your neck. Make sure you let your abs do all the work.

✔ A handful of exercises will help you to work every part of the midsection to create toned, flat abs.

✔ Working the internal and external obliques strengthens and tones your sides.

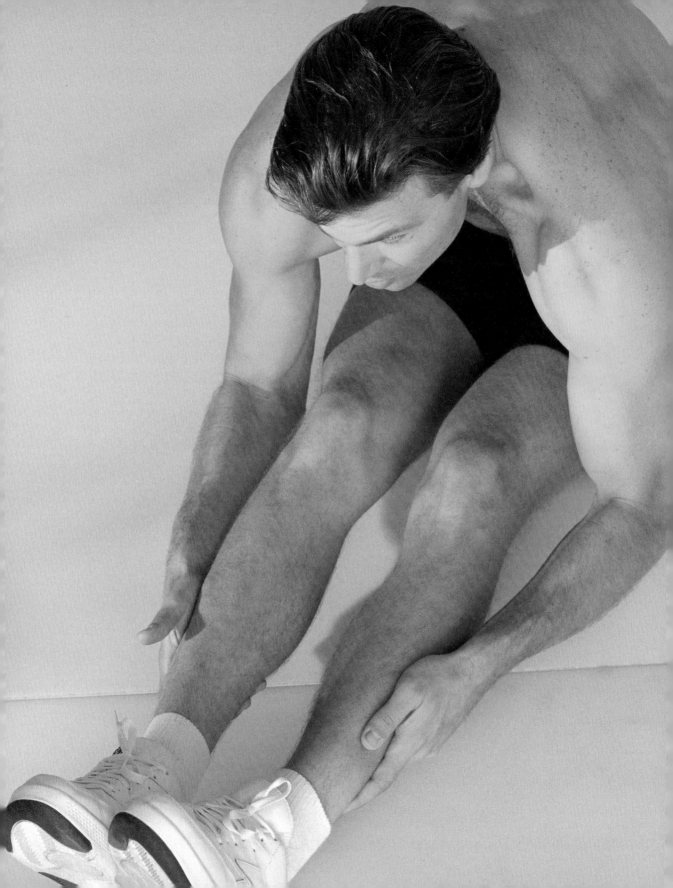

Chapter 13

Lower Body Workout

T HE MUSCLES OF THE LOWER BODY get quite a workout on a daily basis. We use our legs and our rear ends when we walk, sit, jump, stand, or kick. The lower body has the largest muscle groups of the body. Exercise will not only tone these muscles but also increase our endurance. And as an added bonus, firming these large muscles increases our metabolism so that we burn more fat. Read on to learn how to tone and tighten at home or in the gym, and maybe feel better in your favourite pair of jeans.

In this chapter...

✓ Muscles in the lower body

✓ Why you need strong legs and buttocks

✓ Lower body exercises

✓ A few simple exercises with weight machines

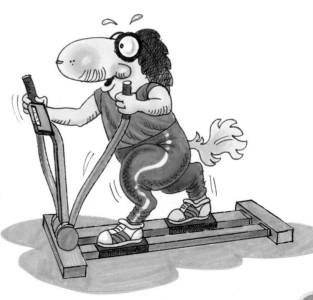

WORKING THE LARGE MUSCLES IN THE LOWER BODY HELPS BOOST YOUR METABOLISM

Muscles in the lower body

THE LOWER BODY is made up of many large muscle groups.
Here are the main muscles that we'll be exercising and toning.

a **Gluteus maximus:** this is the large muscle that spans
across your rear end. This area is usually referred to as
the "glutes." This term can also include the two smaller
muscles of the backside – the gluteus medius above the
gluteus maximus, and the gluteus minimus, which is
below. The gluteus maximus helps straighten your leg
behind you and helps you stand up from a sitting position.
The main job of the gluteus medius and gluteus minimus
is to keep the pelvis steady. You use these muscles when
you walk up hills, stand up from a seated position, climb
stairs, or extend a leg behind you

INTERNET

www.fitnessdirectory.
net/directory/u/
upperleg.html

*For a fuller picture of
muscles in the lower body,
see the excellent detailed
diagram on this page.*

b **Quadriceps:** this large muscle group makes up the front of the thigh.
Sometimes called "quads," it stretches from hip to knee

*The quadriceps are made up of four muscles (quad = four): rectus femoris,
vastus lateralis (outer thigh), vastus intermedius (inner thigh), and
vastus medialis. They are connected by a
common tendon near the knee.*

Since most exercises that work the quads work
all four equally, the four muscles are usually
discussed as one group. The main job of the
quads is to extend and straighten the leg, so
this group of muscles is important for standing,
walking, running, and almost all activities that
involve the legs

c **Hamstrings:** the hamstrings are made up of three
muscles that run down the back of your upper
thigh. These muscles curl or kick the leg back.
(Trust the English language to complicate our
lives. Hamstrings are also tendons at the rear
hollow of the knee; but when we talk about
hamstrings here, we're referring to the muscles)

Trivia...

*The Achilles tendon is the
sinew that attaches the calf
muscles to the back of the
heel bone. It's named after
Achilles of Greek mythology.
When Achilles was a baby,
his mother held him by the
heel and dipped him in the
River Styx to make him
invulnerable, but the heel
didn't get wet. During the
Trojan War, Achilles was
shot in the heel by an arrow
and was mortally wounded.*

Calves: the calf muscles run along the back of your lower leg. They go from the back of your knee and insert into your heel through your Achilles tendon. The largest muscle of the calf is the gastrocnemius, and a smaller muscle of the calf is the soleus

The basic function of the calves is to extend and flex the foot and bend the knee. You use calf muscles when you walk, run, jump, or stand on your toes.

Tibialis anterior: this muscle runs along the front of the lower leg, next to the shin. It runs from the front of the ankle, up alongside the shinbone, up to just below the kneecap. You use this muscle when you lift the front of your foot up while your heel is on the ground

Why you need strong legs and buttocks

THE GOOD NEWS *about exercising the lower body is that you not only tone and strengthen, you also build endurance. The lower body has such large muscles that working them can be an aerobic activity as well as a strengthening one. Also, toning these large muscles raises your metabolism (muscles burn more calories than does fat), so you're burning off fat from your body, even when you're at rest.*

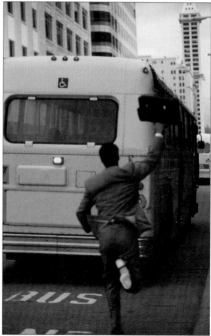

The leg muscles are the strongest and largest group of muscles in the body; they support your weight when you run, jump, walk, or do almost any activity. Since you use these muscles all the time, keeping them in shape can really increase your overall fitness.

■ **Strong leg muscles** *are a real asset when you need to break into a run, such as when sprinting for the bus.*

Lower body exercises

HERE ARE EXERCISES DESIGNED to target the muscles in the lower body. Some of them are multi-muscle exercises, and others focus more on a particular area. You can do all of these without any equipment, but some have a modified version for which you need a chair or something to hold onto, and some require hand weights for a bigger challenge.

Squats

Muscles worked: glutes, quads, and hamstrings.

1 To do a squat, find a comfortable stance with your feet hip-width apart and your toes facing forward or turned slightly out. Never point toes inward. Keep your torso upright and your tailbone pointed down.

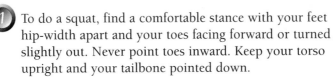

To get a feel for the proper position, try this: tilt your pelvis under, then arch it back. Now, find the spot in the middle.

Your hands can be either on your hips or on your thighs. Focus on something out in front of you; this will help you balance

2 Bend your knees and drop your hips down, sinking your weight into your heels until your hips are almost parallel with your knees. Think about sitting back as if you were going to sit in a chair. Avoid dropping your hips below your knees, pushing your knees forward over your toes, or rolling your knees inward or outward

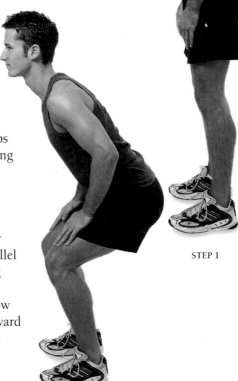

STEP 1

STEP 2

3 Keep your abs tight, and come back up. Make sure to squeeze your glutes extra hard on the upward phase

4 Try 15 reps, or as many as you can do

Modified version: if you have any trouble with the squat, try holding onto the back of a chair for the first few times until you get the hang of it.

With weights: once you find squats easy, try adding weight to increase the intensity of the exercise. Hold a dumbbell (hand weight) in each hand, with your arms down by your sides and your palms facing in. Make sure to continue with good form.

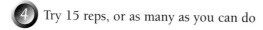

Focus on the muscles you're working while you do squat exercises. Really feel the tension in your rear and thighs.

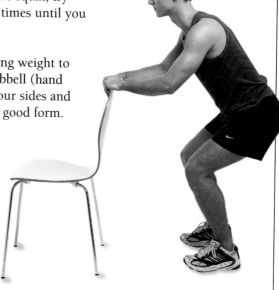

MODIFIED SQUAT

Plié squat

Muscles worked: glutes, quads, and hamstrings.

A *plié* squat is a squat variation that works the inner thigh more. The difference between a plié and a squat is that with a plié you lower straight down using those inner thigh muscles while with a squat you sit back, using the glutes more.

> **DEFINITION**
>
> A **plié** is a ballet move in which the knees are bent while the back is held straight.

1 Spread feet wider than shoulder-width apart and angle them out slightly. Keep your back nice and straight. Again, do not let your knees extend past your toes and don't let your knees flop inside. Be comfortable. Put your hands on your hips

2 Keep abs tight as you drop the centre of your body downwards and perform a deep stretch with your thighs

3 Squeeze with your inner thighs as you come up, keeping the glutes tight

4 Try 15 reps or as many as you can do

Modified version: find a chair (or something else to hold onto) and lightly hold onto the support with both hands while you plié. This is a good way to get the feel for a plié squat, especially if you're having trouble balancing.

With weights: try this while holding a hand weight in each hand. Keep your posture nice and tall, hold weights with palms in, elbows slightly bent, and hands on hips.

Lunges

Muscles worked: quads, hamstrings, glutes, and calves. Lunges also work the abs and upper torso.

1. Start with your feet hip-width apart, then move your left leg back a few feet and pick up your rear heel. Tilt your pelvis forward. Keep your toes facing forward and your weight balanced on both feet

2. Bend your right knee while keeping your upper body straight. Keep your torso upright and your abs pulled in to support your spine

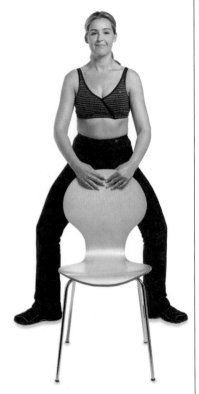

MODIFIED PLIÉ SQUAT

3. Come back up. The movement is akin to going up and down like a horse on a carousel. Your right shin should remain perpendicular to the floor. When you bend your knee, you should feel it mostly in your quadriceps. Your hamstrings and glutes will also be working hard from the action in the hip joint

Keep your chest lifted and abs tight while doing lunges; don't slump.

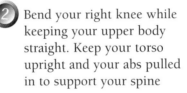

4. Start with 12 reps on one side, then switch legs and repeat

BASIC LUNGE

Here's an added challenge: alternate legs after lunging. Now instead of going up and down with one leg in front, you bring the bent leg back and lunge with the other leg. The same rules about position apply (don't slump, keep abs in, and chest lifted). With both versions, don't let your knee go over your ankle while you're lunging.

Modified version: same as above, but hold onto a support such as a chair, the wall, or a bar. Hold the support at arm's length. Try it like this a few times and get comfortable with the movement before moving on.

With weights: this is the same exercise but with hand weights. You don't need heavy weights, just a bit more resistance. Feel the interplay between your other lower body muscles and your glutes. Hold the weights in your hands, arms down by your sides, palms in. Start with one to two sets of 10–12 reps. Switch legs and repeat.

LUNGE WITH WEIGHTS

Leg extensions

Muscles worked: hamstrings, glutes, quads, and calves.

Leg extension

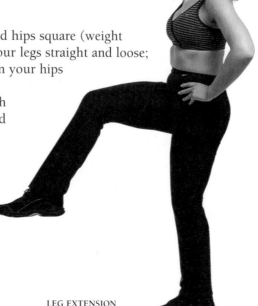

1. Stand up straight, with your abs tight and hips square (weight balanced on both sides equally). Keep your legs straight and loose; don't lock your knees. Put your hands on your hips

2. Lift your right knee up so that your thigh is parallel to the ground, and then extend your toe out

3. Hold here for a beat, then lower right leg back down so that you are back in a neutral standing position. Movement should be slow and controlled all the way up and down. Work on lifting that leg high

4. Work up to doing 20 reps; then repeat with the other leg

LEG EXTENSION

Leg rear extension

1 From the same starting position as the leg extension, place your left heel behind your right, left toes pointing out to the side. Again, knees should be slightly bent, not locked

2 Squeeze your glutes as you lift your left leg behind you as high as you can without straining

3 Hold at the top for a beat, then bring it back down, slowly and with control. These are tight, little squeezes. Keep your hips square, fighting the natural tendency to turn your hips a bit sideways. You will feel this in the glutes

4 Work up to doing 20 reps; then repeat with the other leg

Modified version: if you're having trouble with either the leg extension or the rear extension, put one hand on the back of a chair for balance.

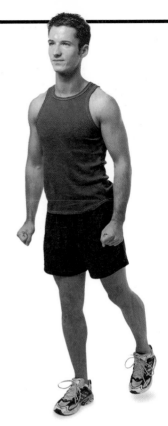

LEG REAR EXTENSION

Single leg curl

Muscles worked: hamstrings.

1 Get down on the floor or mat on your hands and knees, then lower down to your elbows, making sure your elbows stay directly under your shoulders. Keep your back straight and your abs pulled in tight

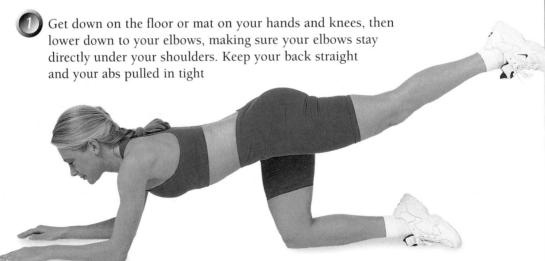

SINGLE LEG CURL

2 Keeping the knee bent, lift one foot toward the ceiling until the thigh is parallel to the floor. Squeeze your buttocks and press the foot slightly higher towards the ceiling

3 Lower and straighten the leg so the thigh is again at hip level, and repeat with the same leg. Make sure you keep thigh at hip level when you lower; don't let your toes touch the ground. Also, keep your weight equally balanced on your elbows and knee. Resist the natural tendency to lean away from the leg you're lifting

4 Do 12 reps on one side; then repeat with the opposite leg

Calf raises

Muscles worked: calves (gastrocnemius and soleus muscle).

Standing calf raise

1 Stand with arms straight down by your sides. Place the balls of your feet on a 2.5–7.5 cm (1–3 in) platform to increase the range of motion of muscles being worked. You can do this on the bottom stair, or a step machine, or any other platform that can support your weight

2 Start with your heels on the ground and lift up your body to the point where you are standing on your toes

3 Briefly hold the contraction, and gently lower your heel to the starting position. The entire movement, which should last about 3 seconds, should be deliberate and controlled. The only movement should occur at the ankle joint. As always, keep those abs tight, chest open, and spine neutral (don't arch your back)

Don't bounce at the bottom or the top of the movement. Always go slowly and stay in control.

4 Work up to 20 reps

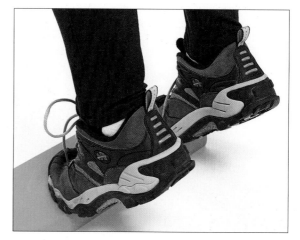

STANDING CALF RAISE

213

Modified: do the same motion without a platform, that is, just rise up on your toes, hold, and come back down.

With weights: hold the dumbbells with palms in and arms straight down by your sides.

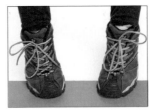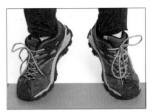

■ **With calf raises,** *you can stand with your toes pointed slightly in for development of outer calf; or widen your feet and bring your heels together for inner-calf development.*

Seated calf raise

1. Sit on a chair or bench with your knees bent at a 90-degree angle

2. Put the balls of your feet on the edge of a ledge, block or step – something about 2.5–7.5 cm (1–3 in) high. Your toes should be pointed forwards

3. Lower your heels as far as possible or until you notice a good stretch in your calves. Then, raise your heels as high as possible. Focus on making your calves do all the work and hold for a few seconds

4. Work up to 20 reps

With weights: for a more challenging seated calf raise, try it with weights. The action is the same, but hold your dumbbells or a weight plate, if you have one, in your lap, near your knees.

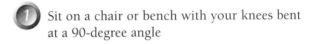

SEATED CALF RAISE

A few simple exercises with weight machines

MANY WEIGHT MACHINES commonly found in gyms can help you target and tone the muscles of your lower body. (For the lowdown on weight machines, see Chapter 3.) Although there are plenty of weight machines and variations on how to use them, here are a few basic gym-specific moves for working the muscles in your lower body.

Glutes and hamstrings

To tone the glutes and hamstrings, try the machine in which you get on your knees and elbows holding onto a grip at the front of the machine. (There are different names for this kind of machine, depending on the brand.)

1. Either push up on a foot pad at the back of the machine or curl your leg under the padded bar depending upon the model of machine

2. Adjust the weight so that you can barely do 12 reps. If you can do more than that without strain, add a bit more weight. If you can't lift it eight times, then lighten your load

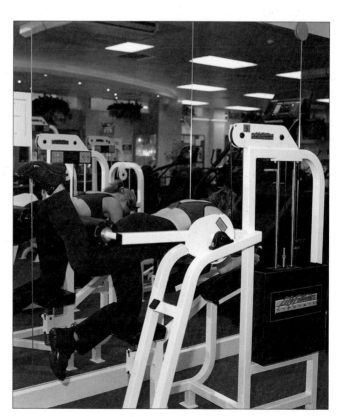

■ **There are many different** *types of glutes machine but they all work the same area.*

Leg press

On this machine the legs press against a weighted platform. The leg press works the quads, hamstrings, and glutes.

1 Place your feet flat on the platform, shoulder-width apart with your toes pointed slightly out. Position yourself so that your knees are at a 90-degree angle

2 Press the platform until your legs are nearly straight. Once again, adjust the weight so that you can barely do 12 reps. If you can do more than that without strain, add a bit more weight. If you can't lift it eight times, then lower the amount of weight

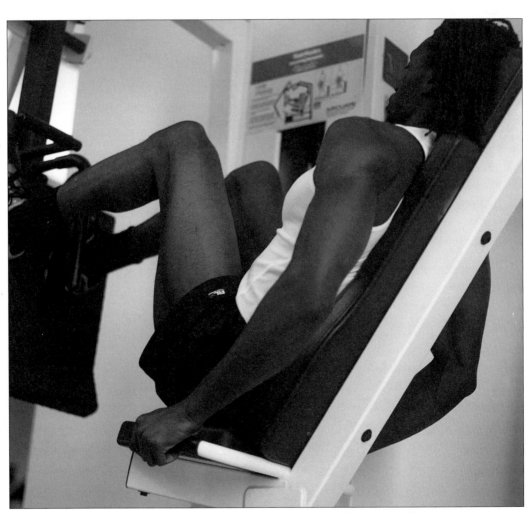

■ **When using the leg press machine,** *you can work your outer thigh more by keeping your feet further apart, and the inner thigh more by keeping your feet closer together.*

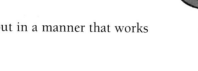

Don't lock your knees or bounce the weight at the top or the bottom of the movement.

Leg press calf raise

This exercise uses the same leg press machine, but in a manner that works the calves.

1. Using the leg press machine, place your toes and the balls of your feet on the edge of the platform so that your heels are up

2. Keep your knees straight, and push the platform by extending your foot (toes higher than heels, calves contracted)

3. Lower the platform by contracting your foot (toes lower than heels, calves stretched). Be very careful not to bounce the weight

4. Repeat until failure or until you have completed the desired number of repetitions – try starting with 12

A simple summary

✔ The main muscles in the lower body are the glutes, quads, hamstrings, and calves.

✔ Working the large muscles in the lower body keeps you in great shape by raising your metabolism while you tone this large muscle group.

✔ Having strong legs makes it easier to get around.

✔ There are plenty of lower body exercises you can do without any equipment.

✔ There are also quite a few lower body workouts you can do on weight machines at the gym.

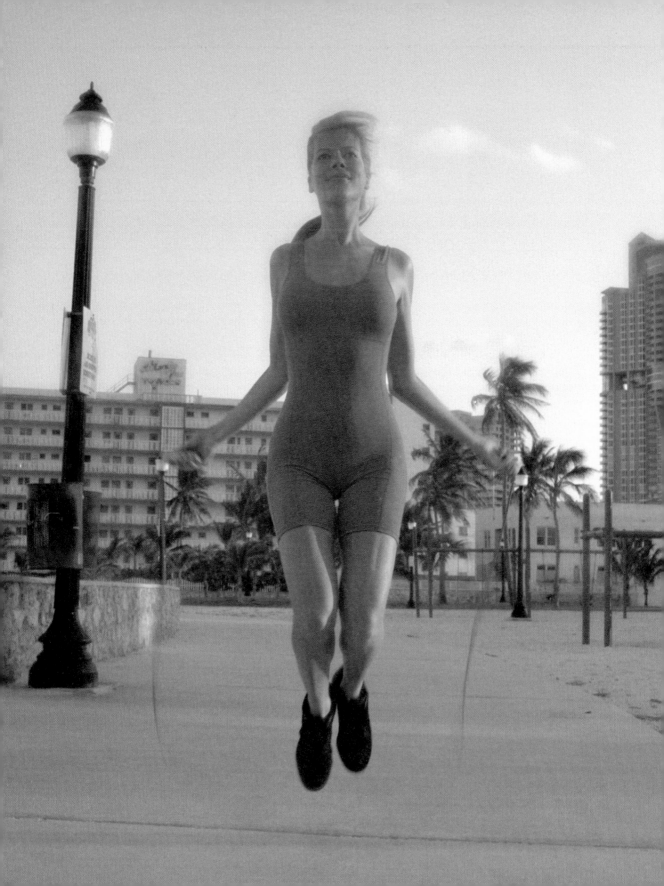

Chapter 14

All-Over Body Quick Fix

B Y NOW WE KNOW WHAT TO DO TO TONE our arms, abs, and legs. But what if you don't have a lot of time and need an all-over body blast? Check out these exercises to work your entire body. We'll do everything from the jumping jacks you remember from gym classes to plyometric training. Don't worry; it's just a matter of jumping and having fun. We'll go through exercises to improve strength, endurance, and mobility – and you don't even need any equipment, just a little floor space.

In this chapter...

✔ Jumping jacks

✔ Skipping

✔ Squat thrusts

✔ Windmill

✔ Plyometrics

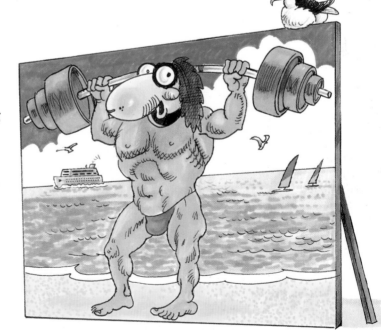

SKIPPING IS GREAT AEROBIC EXERCISE THAT WORKS THE WHOLE BODY

Jumping jacks

AH, OLD FAITHFUL JUMPING JACKS. Maybe you remember these from P.E. lessons. Jumping jacks have been around such a long time because they're effective. They give you a great cardiovascular kick in no time. They're a great way to warm up or to keep up your metabolism during a workout, or they can be a means unto themselves.

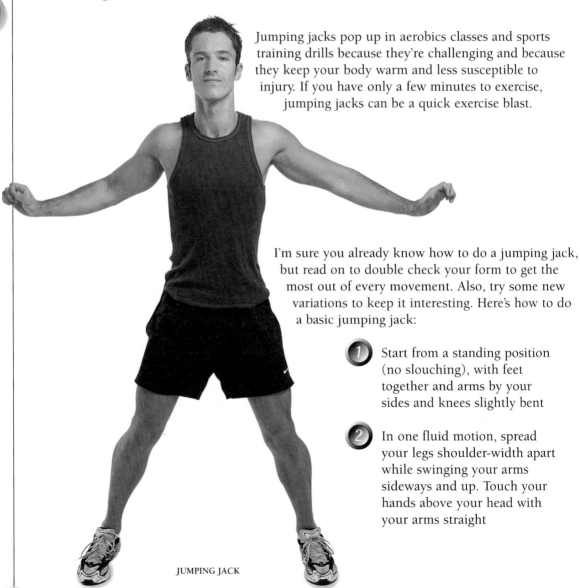

Jumping jacks pop up in aerobics classes and sports training drills because they're challenging and because they keep your body warm and less susceptible to injury. If you have only a few minutes to exercise, jumping jacks can be a quick exercise blast.

I'm sure you already know how to do a jumping jack, but read on to double check your form to get the most out of every movement. Also, try some new variations to keep it interesting. Here's how to do a basic jumping jack:

1. Start from a standing position (no slouching), with feet together and arms by your sides and knees slightly bent

2. In one fluid motion, spread your legs shoulder-width apart while swinging your arms sideways and up. Touch your hands above your head with your arms straight

JUMPING JACK

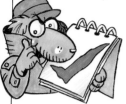

3 Bring your feet back together and your hands to your sides. Ta da! That's one. Try to do them for 2 minutes

To keep it interesting, try doing ten jumping jacks facing one direction, then ten facing another until you come back around to where you started.

JUMPING JACK VARIATIONS

Variation 1: keep your elbows slightly bent throughout the movement so that your hands go from about your belt line to over your head. This gives them a better workout. It brings awareness to your arm muscles and makes you less likely to flop your arms. Keep the tension in your muscles; don't just throw your arms and legs around like cooked spaghetti.

Variation 2: bring your arms straight out from your sides when you hop your legs out, then bring arms and legs down. Next time your legs go out, bring your arms all the way up. Then down, side, down, up and continue for 2 minutes or as long as you can.

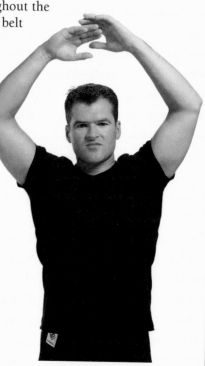

VARIATION 2

Underwater: if you have joint trouble, especially with your knees or ankles, or if you find jumping jacks too jarring, try an underwater jumping jack. Since your body is almost weightless underwater, there's less stress on the joints. At the same time, there is increased resistance to give your muscles a better workout.

Stand in water that's about chest high (water line should be somewhere between armpit and rib cage). Do a jumping jack like the one above, but don't let your arms come out of the water. Also, go slowly and really push. Feel your muscles working against the resistance of the water.

Skipping

SKIP AND FEEL LIKE A KID AGAIN! Jumping through a skipping rope is fun, is a great aerobic workout, and works the entire body. It increases body awareness and develops hand and foot coordination. Before you run outside and **Double Dutch** *with the children down the road, check out these moves.*

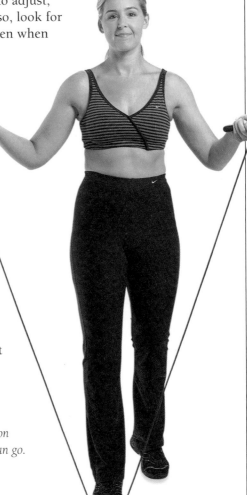

> **DEFINITION**
>
> **Double Dutch** *is an advanced skipping routine in which two rope turners turn and crisscross two ropes.*

Find the right rope

A lightweight, segmented rope is good for beginning and intermediate workouts. Segmented ropes are easy to adjust, and they don't get as tangled as ordinary ropes. Also, look for foam handles because they provide a good grip, even when your hands get sweaty.

Technique

There are endless variations on skipping. Here is a handful to get you started. Make it a game and have fun. See if you can invent your own variations. Aside from the basic two-feet jump, here are other jumping techniques to keep your skipping workout challenging:

Figure eight

This is a good move to start with, to help you get the feel for the skipping rope and the motion before you start jumping. Swing the rope out in front of you and swing it from side to side without jumping through it.

■ **To determine how long** *a skipping rope should be, step on the centre of the rope and pull the handles up as far as they can go. The handles should be around the middle of your chest.*

SKIPPING TIPS

- Wear comfortable shoes with a reinforced toe and lots of cushioning for the ball of the foot. Aerobic or cross-training shoes are good
- Find a good place to jump. An exercise mat, wooden floor, a gym surface, and even carpet are great surfaces for a skipping workout. Concrete is okay, but it's more jarring
- Keep your shoulders relaxed and elbows close to your body
- Bend your knees slightly
- Turn the rope from the wrist, and try to keep a smooth arc in the rope as it passes overhead
- Keep your back straight and head up
- Jump as low as you can (with just enough room to let the rope slide under) to keep the impact on your knees and ankles to a minimum
- Put on some fun, crazy, upbeat music to get you in the mood

There should be no white-knuckled skipping; grip rope handles lightly.

While you're skipping, you can always go back to this move to rest. If you need a break, but you don't want to stop completely, swing the rope by your side until you feel like jumping again.

Double bounce

This is a good move to start your skipping with: jump twice in one rotation of the rope. It's a little easier, and it's a good lead-in to the usual single-bounce jump.

The skier

Instead of jumping straight up and down, keep your feet together and shift them in the air from side to side, as if downhill skiing. You can also keep the rope in your hands and jump from side to side to get a feel for the motion before actually jumping through the rope.

Straddle

This is basically a jumping jack with a skipping rope. This is a more advanced skipping move and again, can be learned by swinging the rope at your side before jumping through it.

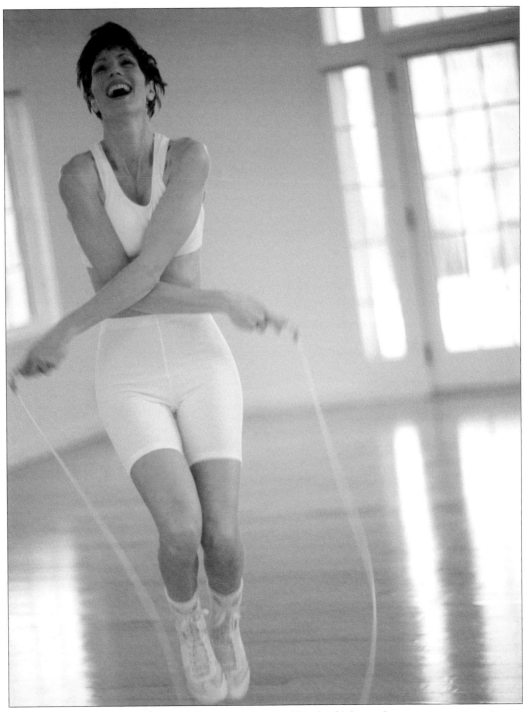

■ **Once you get into the swing** *of skipping, there are all kinds of advanced moves you can experiment with to keep your workouts varied and interesting.*

Slow jump

Cut repetitions in half, elongating the motion. This sounds as if it would be easier, but it's actually more difficult to go slowly like this.

Backwards

Try swinging the rope from front to back. Just be careful not to hit yourself on the head with the rope (not that I would know about that).

High knee

As you jump, bring your knees high. See how far you can get your feet off the ground.

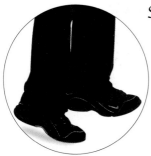

HEEL TAP

Scissors

Scissor your legs back and forth, one leg in front and one in back; then switch. (This is hard.)

Heel tap

Bring one foot out in front, and gently tap your heel to the floor; then repeat with the other foot.

Toe tap

Touch your toe to the floor behind you; then repeat with other foot.

SLOW JUMP

Modification: skip without a rope. If you don't have a rope or if you're not quite up to the challenge, go through the motions without a rope first. I see people doing this all the time in exercise classes. You still get a workout.

Skip for as long as you can. It's hard to keep going for very long. Start by skipping for a few minutes, and work up to more. Aim to skip for 10 minutes.

If you need to take a break, remember that you don't have to stop completely; you can swing the rope to the side for a breather.

If you can skip for 10 solid minutes, you get a prize.

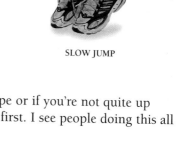

Squat thrusts

ANOTHER BLAST FROM THE PAST, *this exercise gives your cardiovascular system a workout along with your muscles. Glutes, quads, hamstrings, abs, and triceps all get a bit of a workout with this move.*

Basic squat thrust

Start by standing with your feet together. Then drop your hands down in front of your feet, put your weight on your hands, and quickly thrust your legs straight out behind you so that you're in the plank position, like the top of a push-up. In this position, your arms are straight, your body is in one line, and your weight is on your hands and feet. Then, in one quick movement, bring both feet back up behind your hands and return to the standing position. The entire move should be done in a rapid, four-count succession:

1. Down on hands and feet

2. Thrust feet out behind you

3. Bring feet back in

4. Stand up and repeat

Begin with small movements, and increase the movement size as you get more comfortable with the exercise. Here are some variations, starting from the easiest to the most difficult.

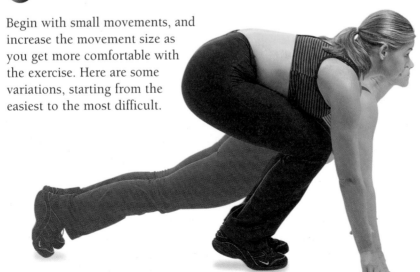
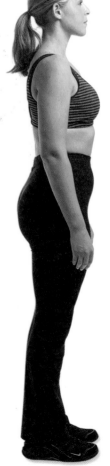

STEPS 1, 2, 3   STEP 4

Modified wall squat thrust

This is a great variation if you are a beginner or if you're just having a low-energy day. From a standing position, place your hands on a solid wall. Place your feet shoulder-width apart, a few feet back from the wall. Lift one knee up towards your chest and put it back down. Then lift the other knee, and continue alternating knees. At first, go slowly and put your foot all the way down on the floor; as you get better, go faster, touching down only briefly on your toes.

Squat thrust without standing

This is the same exercise as the regular squat thrust, but instead of starting in a standing position, you start from the plank position. Start with your hands flat down under your shoulders, facing forward and with your feet together extended behind you.

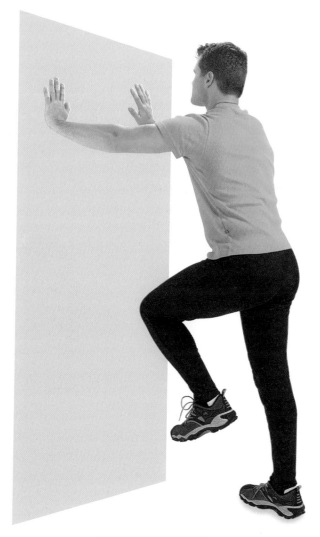

MODIFIED WALL SQUAT THRUST

Staying on your toes, bring both knees up towards your chest. Once your feet have landed up by your chest, thrust them back smoothly to the starting position before repeating.

Alternate leg squat thrusts

Place your hands on the floor, shoulder-width apart, and stretch your legs out behind you in the push-up position. Keeping your left leg where it is, bend your right knee and bring it forward to your chest, as far as is comfortable. In one swift movement, swap the position of your right leg with your left leg. You should now be in a position with your left leg drawn upwards and your right leg stretched out behind you. Continue alternating legs.

Windmill

THIS EXERCISE FEELS GOOD. *It's not quite as challenging as a squat thrust or jumping jack, but it works your body and gives you a good stretch at the same time.*

The windmill challenges the muscles of your trunk, legs, and shoulders, and it enhances your ability to bend and rotate your trunk.

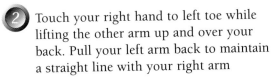

INTERNET

www.benning.army.mil/ usapfs/Doctrine/ calisthenics/cal1-6.htm

This page on the US Army's Physical Fitness School has more information on the windmill plus links to other exercise pages.

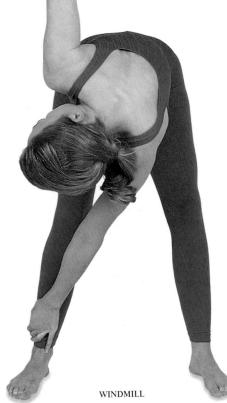

1. Stand up straight, with feet straight ahead, shoulder-width apart. Hips should be square (balanced), abs tight, and shoulders relaxed and down. Arms go straight out to the sides at shoulder height, with palms down. Then bend forward at the waist, and bend your knees slightly

2. Touch your right hand to left toe while lifting the other arm up and over your back. Pull your left arm back to maintain a straight line with your right arm

3. Return to start then repeat, but this time touch your left hand to your right toe. Think about rotating your arms like a windmill

Modification: if you have any upper body difficulties, such as shoulder pain, you can try this with your hands on your hips and do the same movement as above

WINDMILL

Plyometrics

PLYOMETRIC TRAINING *is specific work to enhance explosive power. In other words, it involves a lot of jumping. Plyometric training is used for sports that require short bursts of power such as tennis, basketball, or skiing, but it's also a good exercise for anyone who wants to increase his or her power.*

Have fun

Here are a few plyometric exercises to add to your routine. Once again, I like to think of how people were when they were young – always jumping and hopping around. Apply this attitude of fun and try some jumping. Also, make sure to warm up adequately and stretch before you begin.

Plyometrics is a high-impact activity, so if you have any joint trouble or back pain, give it a miss.

PLYOMETRICS TIPS

- Before a vertical jump, crouch to a point where your knees reach a 90-degree angle
- Use your arms. The inertia of swinging your arms up as you jump will help pull the rest of your body up
- The faster you are moving before the jump, the higher you can jump. This is why high jumpers get a running start – to jump much higher than they could from standing still
- Think about landing with your entire body, not just your feet. The shock of landing is not absorbed by the foot alone; instead it's a combination of the ankle, knee, and hip joints working together to absorb the shock of landing
- Pretend that the ground is hot, and you want to jump back up quickly
- Land quietly. You shouldn't hear a loud slapping noise when your feet hit the ground

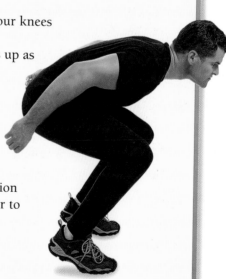

KNEES AT 90-DEGREE ANGLE

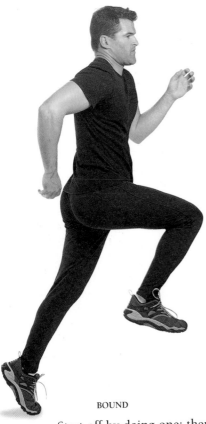

Bounds

Start off by jogging for a few paces. Then push off with your left foot and bring the left leg forward, with knee bent and thigh parallel to the ground. At the same time, reach forward with your right arm. As your left leg comes through, your right leg extends back and remains extended for the duration of the push-off. Hold this extended stride for a moment; then land on your left foot.

Then, the right leg comes through to a forward bent position, the left arm reaches forward, and the left leg extends backward as you continue on the other side. Make each stride long, and try to cover as much distance as possible. You should land on the sole of your foot and immediately take off again. Keep the foot touch-down time as short as possible. Try two or three bounds.

Don't try too many bounds in one go. Quality is much more important than quantity here, especially because these exercises are to build strength and power rather than endurance.

BOUND

Start off by doing one; then work up to doing a maximum of five per set for two or three sets. Always rest between sets.

Single leg hops

Stand on one leg. Push off with the leg you are standing on and jump forward, landing on the same leg. Use a forceful swing of the opposite leg to increase the length of the jump, but aim primarily for height. Land mostly on the ball of your foot, and immediately take off again.

Keep your foot on the ground for the shortest time possible. Try a few times on one side; then try the other. Keep your body vertical and straight. When you start, a straight leg is okay. As you get better, try to pull the heel towards your bottom during the jump.

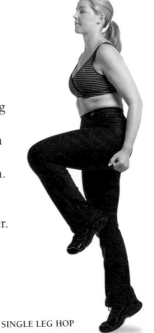

SINGLE LEG HOP

Bunny hops

Stand with your feet shoulder-width apart. Lower into a squat position and jump as far forward as possible. Land mostly on the balls of both feet. Try to keep your body vertical and straight, and don't let your knees move apart or to either side. Use quick double-arm swings and keep landings short.

Tuck jumps

From a standing position, jump up and try to grab both knees up by your chest; this is the ultimate goal, so don't worry if you can't do it right away. It's very challenging.

Return to the starting position, landing mostly on the balls of the feet. Spring up as quickly as you can. Again, try to touch down with your feet very briefly before trying again.

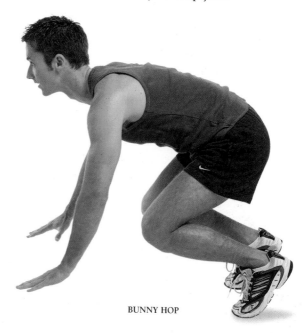

BUNNY HOP

A simple summary

✓ Jumping jacks are a quick way to up your heart rate and tone the muscles. Double check your form to make sure you get the most from your workout.

✓ Grab a skipping rope and act like a child! Skipping is a fun way to get in shape. Adding some new moves can make it more exciting.

✓ Ready to try a squat thrust? If not, check out a few modified versions to help you ease into it.

✓ Loosen up and stay mobile and strong with the all-powerful windmill move.

✓ Jump training, or plyometrics, can increase your strength and power.

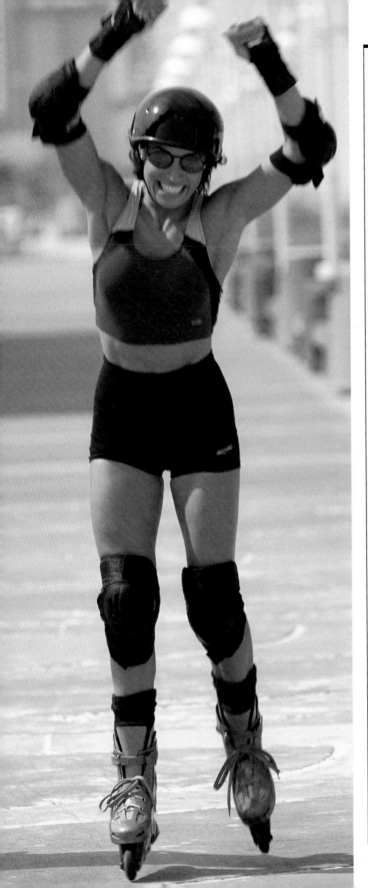

PART FOUR

WITH A FUN REGIME, EXERCISE WON'T FEEL ROUTINE

FITNESS ESSENTIALS

NO FITNESS PLAN IS COMPLETE without *proper nutrition*. Drinking plenty of water and eating a balanced diet are as important to your health as is exercise.

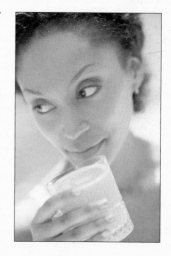

If you are unfortunate enough to sustain an injury while exercising, it doesn't mean you have to give up on your fitness plan. Find out what to do if you *get injured* and how to *know when to stop*. A quick reaction to an injury can prevent serious damage. Do travel plans get you out of your routine? No need to stop exercising. Learn how to get a workout in a hotel room. Or discover the beauty of a fitness adventure, and incorporate some new moves to liven up your workout. Assess your fitness situation: have you been using all three components of a complete exercise programme? Finally, take a peek into the future and learn about upcoming trends in fitness.

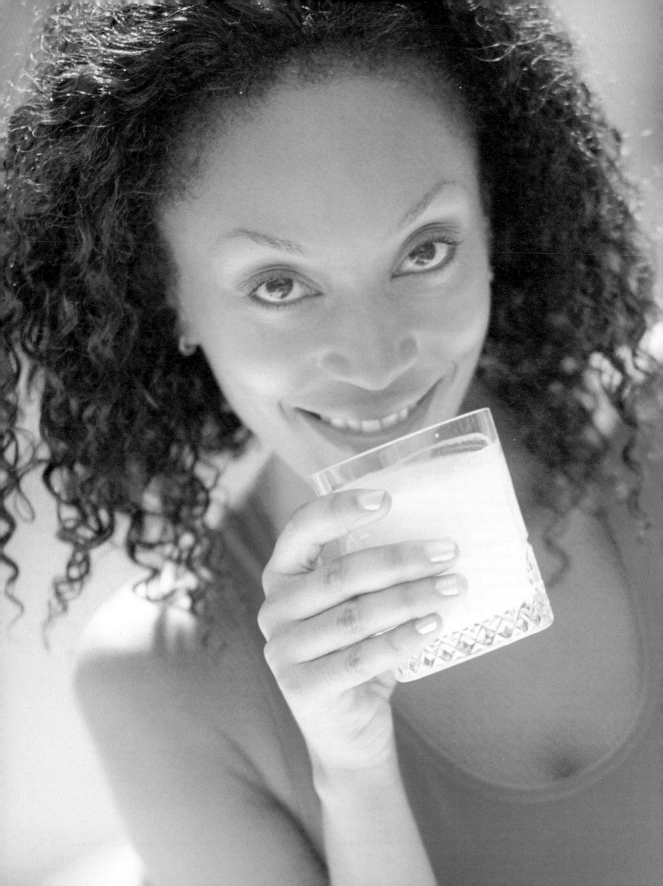

Chapter 15

Simple Nutrition

EATING TO STAY FIT MEANS GOING ON COMPLICATED FAD DIETS or weighing everything on the kitchen scales before eating, right? Wrong! Eating right is a matter of moderation, variety, and balance. Even eating for weight loss doesn't have to be painful. Discover why you need to drink water and how you can tell that you're not getting enough. I'll give you a few tips on healthy eating whether your aim is to lose weight or just to feel better.

In this chapter...

✓ Food and fitness

✓ Water, water everywhere

✓ Healthy eating

✓ Fad diets

✓ Alternative eating

✓ Eat for exercise

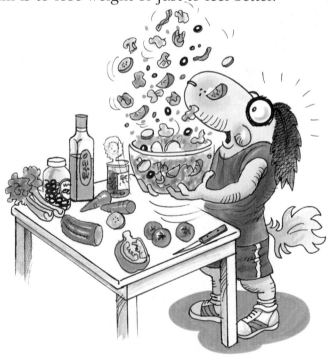

EATING AND DRINKING RIGHT IS AN IMPORTANT PART OF YOUR NEW, HEALTHY LIFESTYLE

Food and fitness

YOU'VE BEEN DOING crunches and push-ups in the mornings before work, you know the people who work at the gym by name, and your running shoes are smoking from overuse. But you can't see the results of your labour. What's wrong with this picture?

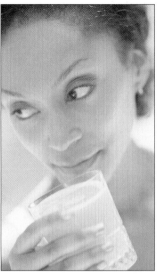

■ **Making the right choices** *about what you eat and drink is key to health and fitness.*

The problem is that you're probably not eating right. In order to really see and feel the results of your exercising, it's important to combine an exercise programme with a smart diet. To put it bluntly, you can't see muscles if they're hidden under a layer of fat. Don't be afraid of the word diet; it merely refers to what you eat. I'm not going to suggest that the only way to get healthy is to eat bark and drink wheat-grass juice.

Eating sensibly

Combining sensible eating with exercise is the best way to get in top shape and to feel healthy. Whether it's weight loss you're after or better health in general, conscious eating can make all the difference. And it doesn't have to be painful or be all about denial. Exercise and good nutrition go together. Just as dieting alone isn't the best way to lose weight, an exercise programme that isn't combined with healthy eating won't be as successful either.

Basically, if you want to lose weight, then you'll need to consume fewer calories than you burn. If you don't wish to lose weight, proper nutrition is still imperative in a healthy and fit lifestyle.

I know people who exercise because they love to eat so much. There's no shame in that. Would you run a mile for chocolate cake? I just might.

■ **Eating healthily** *involves cutting back on high-fat, high-sugar foods and opting for more fresh fruit and vegetables.*

Water, water everywhere

LET'S GET THE EASIEST PART out of the way first – drink water. Most people don't get nearly enough of this precious liquid, yet it is crucial for survival. We should drink at least eight to ten glasses a day. Water is especially important if you're exercising or trying to lose weight. You need to replenish your body with water whenever you exercise and sweat.

Trivia...

The human body is made up of two-thirds water. Virtually every cell in the body needs water. Even our bones are made up of more than 20 per cent water, and our brains and muscles consist of 75 per cent water.

Think you know when you need water because you get thirsty? Well, yes, that's one clue. But many times you're already dehydrated by the time you realize you need water. If your urine is dark or bright yellow, and it's not due to a vitamin you just took, you need more water. That's why you should always have a glass or bottle of water by your side.

The minimum amount of water you should drink in a day is eight glasses, but a general rule is that you need about 15 ml of water per half-kilo of body weight. Therefore, the bigger you are, the more water you should drink. Drink more than that if you're exercising. Also, if you're downing caffeinated or alcoholic drinks, which dehydrate the body, drink an extra cup of water for every soda, coffee, or alcoholic drink you consume.

Order a glass of water whenever you order a beer or even a coffee, and prevent those dehydrators from doing damage. Another perk to drinking water with alcohol is that you'll thank yourself the next morning.

Keep a record

If you're not sure how much water you drink in a day, try this: keep a record of how much water you drink for a few days. Buy a water bottle that holds at least eight glasses, fill it up in the morning, and make sure you've finished it by the time you go to bed.

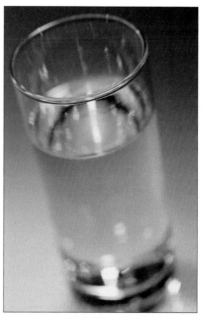

■ **Drinking lots of water** *is good for your health as it helps you lose weight and flushes toxins from the body.*

Drink up

If you're trying to lose weight, water is your best friend. Drink a big glass of water before you eat a meal, and you may find yourself eating less because water acts as a natural appetite suppressant by filling you up. If you're worried about retaining water, drink more. Your body hoards water when you're dehydrated, so giving it more will actually help flush you out. If you usually have canned drink with lunch, try having water instead. It's certainly cheaper (unless you have to buy the fancy bottled water), and it can help you lose weight and keep you hydrated and healthy.

If you replaced one can of fizzy drink a day with a glass of water, you could lose up to 4.5 kilos (10 pounds) in one year.

Healthy eating

THE GOOD NEWS *is that you don't have to obsess over every gram of fat or calorie in every bite of food in order to maintain or get to a healthy weight. This doesn't mean you shouldn't think about fat or calories, it just means that healthy eating doesn't have to involve obsessive diet restrictions.*

If you're eating from all the food groups, you should be able to get all your vitamins and minerals through food without needing supplements. You should consider adding supplements to your diet if you lead a very hectic lifestyle and don't eat right, if you're on a low-calorie diet, if you're a vegan, or if you have dairy allergies. If none of these applies to you, then you should be able to get everything you need by eating a variety of foods.

Simple tips for healthy eating

Some people might need to start out by counting calories and fat just to get the hang of things. This might be necessary for people who desperately want to lose weight and who have had difficulty in doing so. But there are some general tips on healthy eating that can help you lose or maintain a healthy weight without suffering.

 Eat slowly and stop when you're full
This might sound obvious, but many people forget this, especially when they're really hungry. Take your time and chew each bite thoroughly so you're more aware of when you've had your fill. Stop when you're full, even if it means leaving a few delicious bites on the plate

2 Don't over-order

Resist the temptation to order everything that takes your fancy on a restaurant menu. Ask yourself whether you really want a starter, main course, *and* that side order of chips. Choose your meals wisely, and try to avoid dishes that come smothered in sauces. If you must have sauce, order it on the side

3 Recognize the difference between hunger and craving

When you are hungry, eat something. We don't want anyone starving around here. On the other hand, if you're not really hungry but crave a bag of crisps or a jam doughnut, try to find a healthy alternative or go without

4 When an apple just won't do

Sometimes when you really want that doughnut, no number of apple slices is going to help. Go ahead and have a doughnut – *a* doughnut, not three doughnuts. Instead of eating an entire packet of fat-free biscuits, have one real biscuit if that's what you really want, and don't feel guilty about it. Sometimes that's the only way to be satisfied

The magic phrase for eating right is everything in moderation.

5 Variety is the spice of life

Eat a variety of foods every day so you get all the vitamins and nutrients you need. Eat mostly grains, vegetables, and fruits. Cut down on fats, oils, and sweets

6 Arm yourself

Surround yourself with healthy snacks so you're not tempted to eat things that are bad for you. Stock up on apples, bananas, or strawberries for when a sweet tooth hits you. Cut up some carrot sticks, and keep them in the fridge for a quick snack. Apples with a little peanut butter are a great snack

7 Eat small meals

Instead of eating three large meals a day, try eating five or six small meals or snacks throughout the day. This can prevent you from getting really hungry and overeating at mealtime

8 Don't eat just before going to bed

Although I realize this can be difficult because of work schedules, try to have your main meal in the middle of the day instead of at night. Also, eat dinner a few hours before bedtime so you give your body a chance to use some of those calories before you sleep. Because your metabolism slows way down, you don't burn many calories in your sleep. If you do have a late dinner, wash the dishes before you go to bed to burn off a few of those calories before you go to bed

THE FOOD PYRAMID

The food pyramid is a simple graphic tool developed to help people design a healthy diet. It shows the relative proportion of the food groups you should eat every day. The theory is that you should get more of your calories from high-carbohydrate foods and fewer from fat. Medical opinion stands firm: it is easier to store the fat you eat as body fat than it is to store carbohydrates as fat. To increase your carbohydrate intake, eat plenty of sugar-free breakfast cereals, bread, pasta, and rice. Wholegrain varieties are preferable because they contain more vitamins, minerals, and fibre. You should also aim to eat at least five types of fruit and vegetables a day. Choose fresh or frozen fruit and vegetables whenever possible in preference to tinned, and lightly cook or eat them raw to preserve nutrients. Bear in mind that the food pyramid is about eating a balanced diet. It does not necessarily prescribe a low-calorie one. If you overindulge in any of the food groups, you could end up putting on weight as a result.

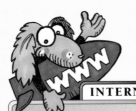

INTERNET

dawp.anet.com

The Diet Analysis Web Page will figure out the amount of calories, protein, and various vitamins and minerals in whatever you eat. Click on the food and the number of servings, enter your gender and age, and back comes a chart or bar graph with the amount of each nutrient and its percentage of the RDA. It includes lots of fast foods by brand.

■ **The food pyramid** *shows the relative proportion of the food groups you should eat every day to ensure a balanced diet. At the bottom, or widest part, are the foods you should eat in the greatest quantities, and at the top are those to be consumed sparingly.*

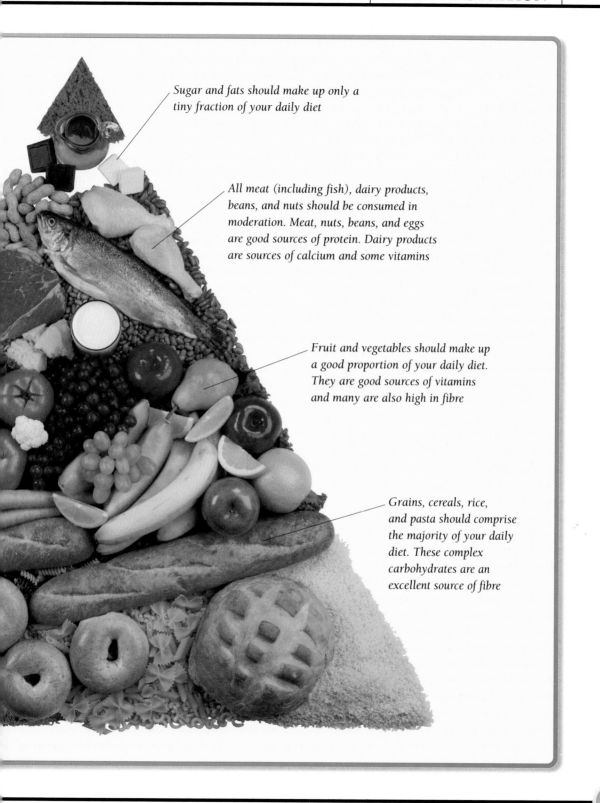

Sugar and fats should make up only a tiny fraction of your daily diet

All meat (including fish), dairy products, beans, and nuts should be consumed in moderation. Meat, nuts, beans, and eggs are good sources of protein. Dairy products are sources of calcium and some vitamins

Fruit and vegetables should make up a good proportion of your daily diet. They are good sources of vitamins and many are also high in fibre

Grains, cereals, rice, and pasta should comprise the majority of your daily diet. These complex carbohydrates are an excellent source of fibre

Calorie counting

Food is made up of calories, also called energy. It's the fuel for your body. The bottom line regarding calories is, if you want to lose weight, consume fewer calories than you use in a day. If the most you've moved all day is to walk to your car and back, then you don't need to eat as much as you would if you had run a 5k (3.1 miles), for example. If you want to maintain your weight, eat as many calories as you burn. And if you need to gain weight, you should eat more calories than you burn in a day. In general, young children, sedentary women, and older folks need about 2,000 calories a day. Active older boys and young men need about 2,400 calories a day to maintain their weight.

Yes, you say, but how do I know how many calories I'm eating? The best way to know what's in your food is to read the labels.

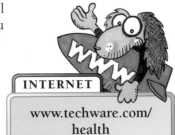

INTERNET

www.techware.com/
health

This is one of a few web sites that will consider your height, weight, age, and lifestyle (active, sedentary) and calculate exactly how many calories you need in a day.

As for knowing how many calories you burn: the exact number of calories a certain activity will burn depends on your size (height and weight), metabolism, and what kind of activity you're doing. In general, aerobic exercise burns the most calories.

Even if you're trying to lose weight, don't consume fewer than 1,200 calories a day.

Cutting down on fat

Fat calories are the most fattening and the most unhealthy. They should be eaten sparingly. That's why over the last few years, hundreds of fat-free and reduced-fat items have hit the market. Before we get into more fat bashing, I should mention that we do need a little fat in our diets. Fat maintains skin and hair, protects cell walls, and keeps our bodies warm. So you don't want to go for a totally fat-free diet. Unsaturated fats, the kind that come from nuts, olive oil, peanut oil, sunflower oils, soya beans, and fatty fish, are the "good" fats. These are the best sources from which to get fat.

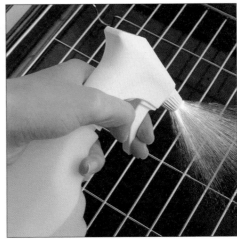

■ **Cut back** *on the amount of fat in your cooking by using a non-stick spray instead of oil.*

Stay away from saturated fats, the kind found in butter, meat, full-fat dairy products, and tropical oils like palm and coconut. Also, stay away from transfatty acids. Transfatty acids are found in solid margarine and vegetable shortening; you're better off using butter.

Too much fat makes us fat and can cause other health problems. If you're eating 2,000 calories a day, you should consume fewer than 65 grams of total fat. These should include no more than 20 grams of saturated fat. And, keep in mind that just because a product is fat-free or low-fat, it still has calories.

Simple ways to cut down on fat:

1. Use low- or non-fat dairy products when cooking

2. Try using a smaller amount of strong flavoured, regular cheese instead of a more lavish amount of mild or low-fat cheese

Cheese is the one dairy product that usually doesn't taste nearly as good when it's low- or non-fat.

3. Toast nuts to bring out the flavour so you don't need as many

4. Use non-stick cooking spray, water, or stock when sautéing. If foods are sticking to the pan, splash a little water in there instead of adding more oil

5. Oil holds taste on the palate, so when you cut down on the oil you use in cooking, increase your use of fresh herbs and spices to compensate

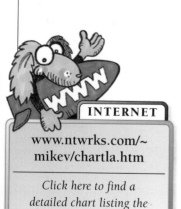

INTERNET

www.ntwrks.com/~ mikev/chartla.htm

Click here to find a detailed chart listing the calorie and fat content of hundreds of foods.

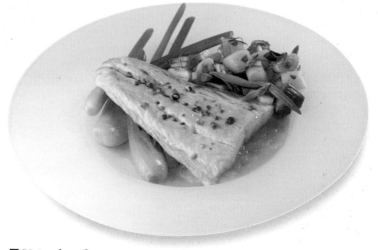

■ **Using less fat in your cooking** *doesn't mean you have to compromise on flavour. Tempt the tastebuds with oil-free sauces, herbs, and spices.*

Fad diets

YOU'RE READY TO MAKE A CHANGEOVER to healthy eating, or maybe you just want to lose weight, and you see an ad for a miracle diet that promises instant weight loss, a fulfilled life, and so on. Don't buy it! Be wary of any diet that offers a quick fix, dictates that entire food groups are off limits, or promises you a new body just by popping pills. Also, watch out for diets that claim to change body chemistry or diets for which you must buy a particular product.

The key to successful weight loss isn't in finding some impossible-to-follow, trendy diet but in making changes you can keep for life. Not only are some of these fad diets hard to follow, some of them are dangerous.

Some of the high-protein, no carb diets will help you lose weight, but as soon as you go back to eating normally, even sensibly, you wind up putting the weight back on. When you block out an entire food group, you're bound to miss out on some important vitamins and minerals. When you cut out carbohydrates, for example, you're not getting enough calcium, fibre, or healthy plant chemicals. And some miracle diet pills have even proven to be deadly.

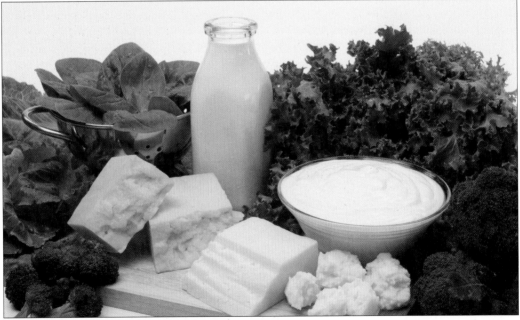

■ **Any diet that advocates** *cutting out entire food groups and concentrating on one or two types of food only is likely to be bad for your health, because you may not be getting all the nutrients you need.*

Alternative eating

IN ADDITION TO FAD DIETS *and other regimens for monitoring food intake, many people choose alternative diets for health, religious, or social reasons. For many, adopting an alternative diet is a matter of personal choice. We're lucky that we can make such choices; in many impoverished parts of the world, you eat what you can! Vegetarianism, and to a lesser extent veganism, is a trend that is gaining in popularity. Another diet that trickles outside the mainstream but is popping up in restaurants and cookbooks is raw foodism, which is just as it sounds – eating only food that hasn't been cooked.*

Vegetarianism

These days, more and more people are going veggie. Some people are cutting down on meat for health reasons; others avoid meat altogether for reasons of health or compassion for animals. Whatever the reason, a *vegetarian* diet is a healthy one.

Vegetarians are usually very healthy people. That might be because many vegetarians also embrace a healthy lifestyle. It is very possible to be a chubby vegetarian; after all chips, biscuits, and chocolate don't have any meat. (I have to admit, though, that I've never met a chubby vegan.) If you make the choice not to eat meat, you just have to make sure that you get enough iron and protein through other sources.

> **DEFINITION**
>
> A **vegetarian** is a person who doesn't eat meat. There are many different kinds of vegetarians. The most common is ovo-lacto vegetarians, who eat dairy and eggs but no meat, fish, poultry, or seafood. Lacto-vegetarians eat dairy but no eggs or meat, fish, poultry, or seafood. Vegans eat no animal products whatsoever.

I became a vegetarian 16 years ago and haven't had any trouble getting all the necessary vitamins and minerals. I have plenty of energy, and I got a thumbs up on my cholesterol levels and blood pressure the last time I went to the doctor.

There are plenty of vegetarian sources of iron, like spinach, raisins, prunes, squashes, black-eyed beans, lentils, chickpeas, and nori (toasted seaweed like the kind that's wrapped around sushi). Vitamin C helps your body absorb iron, so make sure to get enough of that as well. As for protein, I know plenty of people who shy away from a vegetarian diet because they're afraid they won't get enough of the all-mighty protein, but soya products (tofu, tempeh) and many other beans and grains provide plenty of protein.

Raw foods

Some vegetarians have taken it a step further and eat only raw foods. The raw food trend, which started in the US in California, is gaining in popularity. It means what it sounds like – eating only food that hasn't been cooked.

Raw foodists don't eat any food that's been heated to more than 47° C (116° F). The thinking behind this is that cooking foods destroys the natural enzymes.

So why do they do it? Raw foodists believe that food was made to be eaten raw and that cooking it prevents us from gleaning all the nutrients we can out of food. They believe that nature has combined all the nutrients we need in perfect harmony, and so we don't need to alter it. What do I think? I think it's important to include a lot of raw foods in your diet. We can learn a lot about food by acknowledging these trends even though they may seem a little extreme. Remember the watchwords: everything in moderation.

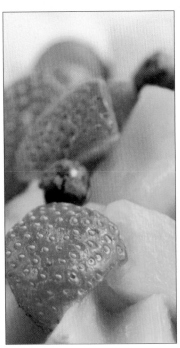

■ **Raw foods** *are packed with nutrients, so it's a good idea to include plenty of them in your diet.*

Eat for exercise

NUTRITION AND EXERCISE go hand in hand. If you're exercising a lot, you want to make sure to get the right kind of fuel in your body for optimal performance. Hardcore athletes often have particular food rituals, like runners who load up on carbs the night before a marathon with a giant pasta dinner. But for general fitness, we just want to get enough fuel for maximum energy for the workout, but not so much food that we're weighed down or get a cramp or stomachache. So, the best thing to do is wait 2 hours after a big meal before working out, but don't hit the gym on an empty stomach.

If you're starving, have a light snack like a banana or an energy bar half an hour before you exercise. Some people recommend having half a bagel (or other piece of bread with nothing on it) and half a cup of coffee before exercising to get a carb and caffeine pick-me-up. If you're hungry immediately after the workout, help yourself to a protein shake or protein bar and have a good meal a couple of hours later. It's hard to fit this in, but if possible, wait 2 hours before and 2 hours after exercising to have a big meal.

Also, water is especially important when you're exercising. Drink plenty of water 2 hours before, immediately before, during, and after your workout to stay properly hydrated.

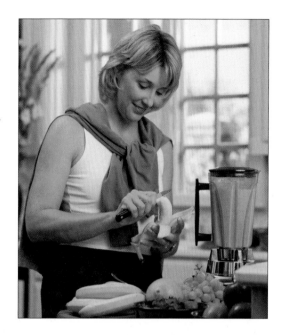

■ **A fruit or protein shake** *will help fill the gap if you feel hungry immediately after a workout.*

A simple summary

✔ You can exercise all you like, but if you aren't eating right you're not going to reap the many benefits of having a healthy body.

✔ Did you know that by the time you're thirsty you're already dehydrated? Drink up! (Drink up the water, that is.)

✔ Cutting down on fat and calories (combined with exercise) is the best way to lose weight. This doesn't mean you can never eat another biscuit. Smart eating means everything in moderation.

✔ Don't be seduced by unhealthy fad diets that promise unrealistic weight loss.

✔ Everyone has eating hang-ups, some of which are healthier than others. Vegetarians don't eat meat, and raw foodists don't cook anything.

✔ Food is the fuel that can propel you through a workout.

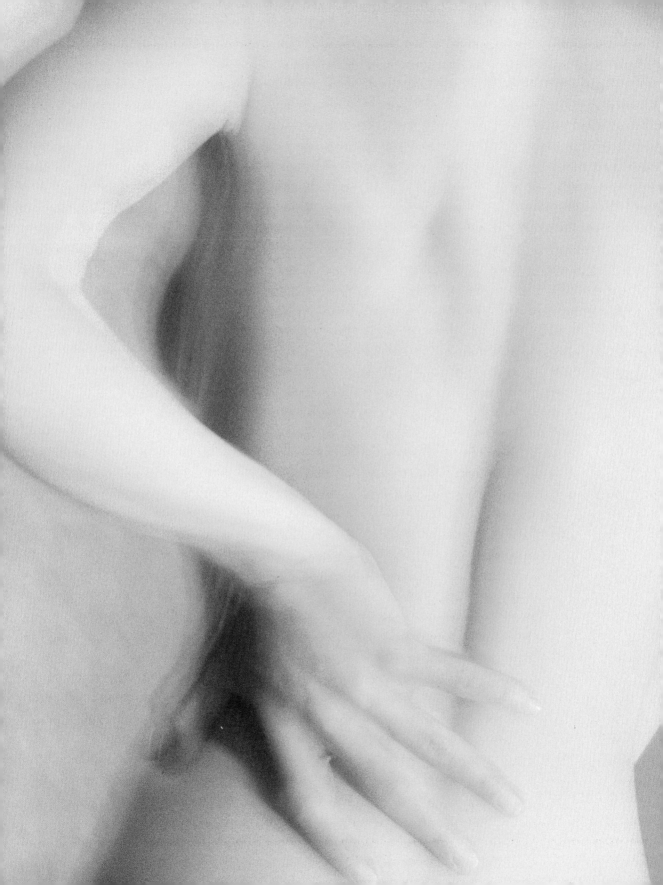

Chapter 16

Special Needs and Injuries

EXERCISE DOESN'T HAVE TO HURT to be effective, but what should you do if it does? Discover what kind of pain is normal and what kind of pain means: "Stop immediately!" Learn what to do if you get injured and how to prevent it from happening again. We'll look at massage and how it can help get you back in the gym, relieve stress, or just make you feel thoroughly pampered. Finally, we'll take a quick look at what exercises you can do if you're pregnant.

In this chapter...

✓ Ouch! Was that supposed to hurt?

✓ Treatment, recovery, and prevention

✓ Massage

✓ Working out while pregnant

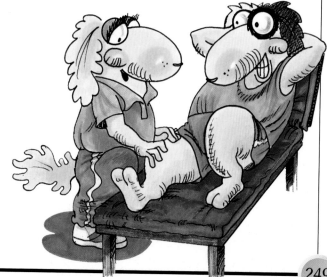

IF YOU FEEL PAIN, IT'S IMPORTANT TO SEEK TREATMENT IMMEDIATELY

Ouch! Was that supposed to hurt?

A LITTLE SORENESS *can be expected when participating in an exercise programme. There are some pains, though, that could indicate an injury that needs to be treated. Muscle soreness is okay, but a pulled muscle is not. Knowing the difference can save you a lot of pain and recovery time. Catching an injury in the early stages can help keep the damage to a minimum.*

Muscle soreness = good pain

Exercising doesn't have to hurt to be effective, but a few aches do come with the territory. Muscle soreness is acceptable. You can recognize muscle soreness when your muscles feel heavy or burn a bit during a workout or start aching a few hours later and perhaps ache the next day. This type of delayed onset soreness is not harmful and is to be expected when you up the intensity of your workout.

But do remember what I told you about muscle soreness back in Chapter 10: don't exercise muscles that ache. Give them at least 48 hours to recover before you work them again. Working muscles when they are sore increases your likelihood of injury. Alternate your workouts, such as exercising your upper body one day and your lower body the next, to give muscle groups a little rest.

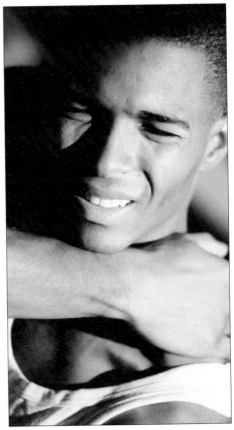

■ **A little muscle soreness** *is to be expected if you're exercising properly – what's important is to take sufficient time to recover.*

If you're sore after a workout (but not injured), a hot shower or a soak in a hot bath can feel really good.

Sprains, pulls, and other injuries = bad pain

Any time you feel a sharp pain, you feel pain immediately after a workout, the pain is worse on one side of the body, or it doesn't go away in 48 hours, you might have a pulled muscle or other injury. A pulled muscle can feel like a tear when it happens, and it hurts a lot even when you stop. You feel muscle strain, have restricted range of motion, and feel stiffness and pain.

When you injure the ligaments that connect bones to one another, you have a sprain. When you get a sprained ankle, for example, you've injured the ligaments around the ankle.

If you think you have an injury, see your doctor.

Here are some other common sports injuries to look out for:

Stress fractures of the foot

What it is: these are small cracks in the bones of the foot that often develop from excessive impact.

What it feels like: pain in the front part of the foot that starts hurting during a long workout, then feels better when you stop. Next time you work out, the pain comes earlier and lasts longer even when you stop.

How to avoid it: wear sturdy, supportive athletic shoes. People with high arches are susceptible. Also, a sudden increase in exercise can bring this on, so increase your exercise intensity gradually.

I have a friend who discovered the joy of step classes and went 7 days a week, until she was grounded with a stress fracture in her foot.

Shin splints

What it is: this is muscle damage along the side of the shin.

What it feels like: ouch. I've had these – they really hurt. They're a drag because they often happen to both legs at the same time, so you don't know which leg to limp on (resulting in occasional mockery by fellow exercisers). The pain runs along the front and outside of the shin after the heel strikes the ground when running or inside the lower leg when you go up on tiptoes.

How to avoid it: once again, get supportive shoes. Also avoid running on banked surfaces, and warm up and stretch before running.

Achilles tendinitis

What it is: this is an inflammation of the Achilles tendon. It happens when too much stress is placed on this tendon.

What it feels like: it hurts! You feel pain behind the heel when you start moving after being still or when you start to run or jog.

How to avoid it: you guessed it – get some good, supportive shoes. Also, be careful when running up or down hills, and try not to land too far back on your heel. Although this injury can start to feel better when you start exercising, because the area gets warm and pliable, it's important to refrain from running or riding a bike until your Achilles tendon heals. Otherwise, you could develop permanent scar tissue that will make that area continue to hurt.

Runner's knee

What it is: the kneecap rubs against the thighbone when the knee moves.

What it feels like: you feel pain, and sometimes swelling under the kneecap starts while you're running. At first, running downhill hurts. Later any running or walking down steps is painful.

How to avoid it: this is usually caused by structural problems, but you can reduce your chances of getting runner's knee by strengthening your thigh muscles and by warming up and stretching thoroughly before running.

■ **Runner's knee** *causes pain and sometimes swelling.*

Forehand tennis elbow

What it is: you don't have to play tennis to get this one. This is a result of damage to the tendons that bend the wrist towards the palm.

What it feels like: pain on the palm side of the forearm from the elbow towards the wrist.

How to avoid it: forehand tennis elbow is caused by bending the wrist towards the palm with excessive force, like when you hit a tennis forehand, or throw a cricket ball, or even carry a heavy suitcase. With tennis, avoid hitting wet balls or using a racket that's too heavy or a grip that's too small. And learn to pack lightly.

Backhand tennis elbow

What it is: backhand tennis elbow is damage to the tendons that bend the wrist backward away from the palm.

What it feels like: it hurts on the outer, back, and side of the forearm.

How to avoid it: this damage generally does come from hitting a backhand in tennis. Using bad backhand form, playing with a racket that's too short or strung too tightly, and hitting heavy, wet balls all contribute to getting this injury. Get a good racket, and have someone check your backhand form.

When to work through and when to take a break

Pain = no gain. Stop exercising the moment you feel any pain (not just a little aching). If you stop right away, you limit the injury and speed up your recovery time. If you continue to work out, you could tear more muscle fibres, causing more damage and delaying your recovery.

Other signals that you should cut your workout short are feeling any pain or pressure in the left or mid-chest area, left neck, shoulder, or arm during or just after exercising. This could be a sign of heart trouble. Also, if you feel light-headed all of a sudden, or if you break out in a cold sweat, or even faint, stop exercising and call a doctor.

Don't worry if you get a stitch; a pain below your bottom ribs is not the result of a heart problem. Getting a stitch in your side sometimes happens when you exercise vigorously. It's nothing to be alarmed about.

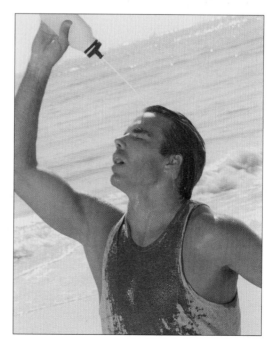

■ **If you are exercising** *in the heat, be careful to avoid heat stroke, which makes you feel dizzy, weak, and very tired. Another symptom of heat stroke is that you stop sweating. Stop exercising and find some shade or other cool place if you experience any of those symptoms.*

Treatment, recovery, and prevention

THE FIRST THING TO DO *with a sports injury is to apply RICE. No, I don't mean slapping a spoonful of rice on your leg.*

RICE stands for Rest, Ice, Compression, and Elevation.

Rest the injured part immediately to minimize internal bleeding or swelling and to prevent the injury from getting worse. That means: don't finish the squash or tennis game first; stop and sit down to avoid further damage. Next, apply ice to the injured area. You can use an ice pack, or crushed ice in a bag, or even a bag of frozen veggies. Place a towel between the skin and the ice to lesson the cold shock a bit. Hold the ice in place for at least 10 minutes. For compression, wrap the area with an elastic band. You can keep the ice in place with this. And keep the injured area elevated. Ice causes the blood vessels to constrict, reducing swelling and pain. Ice should be kept on the injury for 10 minutes and removed for 10 minutes. This process can be repeated several times for the first day.

There has been a lot of controversy over when to apply heat. A few years ago, specialists said to apply heat right away; now they say to apply ice. The general consensus now is not to apply heat for at least 48 hours after an injury. I recommend avoiding heat for injuries. But applying heat to stiff and sore muscles is okay.

Some over-the-counter remedies for soreness and pain are good old ibuprofen, which can reduce pain and swelling, and the herb *Arnica montana*. Arnica is a herb that's popular for pulled or strained muscles. It comes in gel or tablet form, and it reduces inflammation, decreases pain, and some swear it speeds up recovery time.

Recovering from an injury

If you have suffered an injury, avoid participating in whatever sport or exercise you were involved in at the time until your injury has healed. This doesn't mean you have to gaze longingly out of the window while everybody else has fun; it just means you have to find a substitute activity. If you got shin splints playing football, then try swimming or even Pilates. Give yourself a break and don't rush back into anything. You could risk making your injury worse. Wait until the pain disappears before you get back into the activity that caused the injury.

Prevention

The best thing, of course, is to not get injured in the first place. To avoid injury, let me remind you of some basic rules:

1 Schedule strenuous workouts at least 48 hours apart

2 Train gradually

3 Strengthen your muscles with resistance training

4 Warm up, stretch, and cool down with every exercise session

Massage

THE PURPOSE OF MASSAGE *is to alleviate stress and tension that can build up in your soft tissues — your muscles, tendons, and ligaments. Massage has been around forever, but is being used increasingly for sports therapy. Massage is good for athletes with pulled muscles or soreness, people with aching backs or other aching parts, and people who are stressed out. If you've never had a massage, treat yourself and schedule one.*

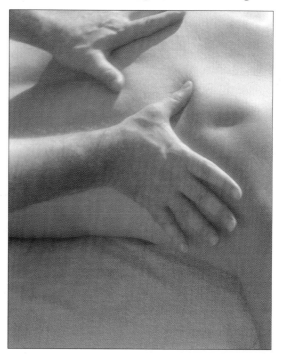

I really love getting a massage, but the first few times I got them they weren't so great. I just didn't feel comfortable with a male massage therapist at first, so I could never totally relax. Since those first awkward times, I've had female and male therapists, and I've enjoyed the massages immensely. Find out about where and from whom you're getting a massage, and don't be shy about requesting a male or female. It's important that you feel completely comfortable.

■ **A relaxing massage** *can revitalize both body and soul, relieving the stresses and strains of the day and soothing tired or aching muscles.*

For some massages you can take off your clothes or wear a swimming costume or trunks – especially if you're having a hydra massage, which involves water. If you're not sure, just ask. If you'd feel more comfortable in your swimming gear or underwear, wear that. Also, drink lots of water after you get a massage because massage is detoxifying. It gets your circulatory and lymphatic systems moving, and flushes out toxins. With this rapid cleansing, it's important to stay hydrated with plenty of water. Otherwise you may feel dehydrated and get a headache.

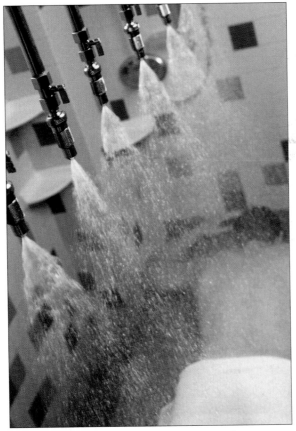

■ **Hydra massage** *involves using water to relieve tension and muscle inflammation. Jets of water are also thought to help stimulate the circulation and internal organs.*

INTERNET

www.massagenetwork .com

Click here for information on different kinds of massage, what to expect from a massage, and how to find a therapist in your area.

Different types of massage

Here are descriptions of some commonly offered massages:

Sports massage: this can help enhance an athlete's performance, prevent injury, and promote recovery. It focuses on the muscles relevant to the particular athletic activity. Even if you aren't an "athlete", this kind of massage feels really good, especially after a big workout.

DEFINITION

In Chinese philosophy, the **meridians** *are channels in the body that the chi, or life force, flows through.*

Shiatsu massage: normally done fully clothed, this involves pressing points on the body, and stretching and opening the energy *meridians*. Shiatsu is a little like acupuncture without the needles. Its proponents view it as a form of treatment alternative to medicine or surgery.

Stone therapy: in this type of massage, hot and sometimes cold stones are used along with regular massage (using hands). Stones are used as massage tools and are also placed all over the body such as between toes, on the forehead, or along the spine. Each treatment is individualized according to where you have stress or pain. The stones allow for a deeper massage, and the heat therapy aids relaxation.

Swedish massage: this involves applying pressure to deep muscles and bones and rubbing in the same direction as the flow of blood returning to the heart. Swedish massage can relax muscles, increase circulation, and give you a better awareness of your body and the way you move. Swedish massage shortens recovery time from muscular strain by flushing metabolic wastes out of the tissues. It stretches the ligaments and tendons, keeping them supple. It's great for general stress relief.

Chair massage: this is one name for a short (15–20 minute) massage for which you sit in a special, portable massage chair on which you put your face down. You remain clothed. No oils are used while your shoulders, neck, upper back, head, and arms are massaged. This is the kind of massage that some large companies provide as a perk for their employees. Sometimes, chair massage booths are set up in busy shopping centres, providing a welcome respite if you've shopped 'til you feel you could drop!

Manual lymphatic drainage: this healing technique blends soothing, gentle, rhythmical, precise, massage-like movements to accelerate the flow of lymphatic fluid in the body. Despite the fancy name, it feels really good.

Deep tissue massage: this is used to release chronic muscle tension through slower strokes and more direct pressure or friction applied across the grain of the muscles. It's an invigorating experience that's a process of finding the stiff or painful areas by feeling the quality and texture of the deeper layers of musculature and slowly working into these deep layers of muscle tissue. Sometimes the therapist will encourage breathing and movement to release and relax muscles.

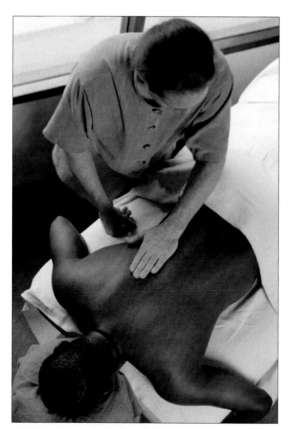

■ **Massage therapy** *should be an agreeable and soothing experience. If you feel any discomfort, tell the practitioner, who can ease the pressure.*

Working out while pregnant

REMEMBER THE DAYS *when pregnant women were not supposed to do anything, much less exercise? Well, those days are over. Not only is it allowed, pregnant women are encouraged to do a little exercise. Whether you have a fitness routine firmly in place or you want to be a bit healthier for the wee one, exercising while pregnant can make you feel great.*

Exercising during pregnancy is good for you for all the same reasons it's good for everyone else. Furthermore, it can help you carry that extra weight around, physically prepare you for the stress of labour, and make it easier to get back in shape after the baby is born.

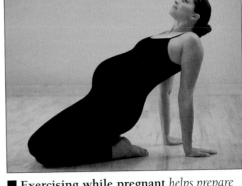

■ **Exercising while pregnant** *helps prepare you for labour and keep you in good physical shape. The golden rule is not to overdo it.*

Having said that, let me add that you should always check with your doctor or midwife about exercising while pregnant. And, this is not the time for any strenuous training; this is the time to enjoy a few mellow workouts.

Keep it low-impact

Some pregnancy-friendly exercises include: walking (great stress relief, low-impact); swimming (works big muscle groups, and you get to be weightless); cross-country skiing (if you fall, at least you don't fall down a mountain); low-impact aerobics (you keep one foot on the floor at all times). Don't even think about horse riding, downhill skiing, water skiing, surfing, or cycling. These are bad news because pregnancy throws your balance off, and you don't want to risk taking a major spill with the little one.

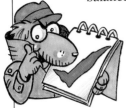

I find tennis on lots of "do" and "don't" lists about exercising while pregnant. My mother played tennis until her seventh month with me, and everything came out okay. (Just wish I could've inherited her killer serve.)

The bottom line is, exercise moderately and don't push yourself too hard. If you're in pretty good shape and you want to play a nice game of doubles, go ahead. Just don't start training for Wimbledon when you're pregnant.

Exercise tips for pregnant women

Here are a few other cautions to keep in mind:

① Stay off your back. After the first 3 months, avoid exercise that requires you to lie on your back for long periods. This restricts blood flow to the fetus. Also, avoid standing for long periods

② Don't hyperventilate. No need to breathe very heavily now. If you start to feel yourself breathing heavily, take it down a notch. Slow down

③ Be aware of balance problems. Your centre of gravity shifts during pregnancy, so avoid activities in which you risk falling

④ Eat. You have the green light to eat more when you're pregnant – about 250 calories a day more. Add on a few extra if you're exercising

⑤ Don't overheat. You're already generating lots of extra heat, especially in the first 3 months. If you feel yourself getting too hot, relax, have some water, find a cool place to sit

⑥ Don't overstretch. Your joints are extra loose when you're pregnant, so be careful not to stretch too far. The joints stay loose for about 4 months after delivery, so be aware of that after the baby is born

Trivia...

Morning sickness is a good thing? According to a recent study, the nausea and vomiting so many women experience during the first few months of pregnancy may actually nourish the baby by keeping certain hormone levels in check.

A simple summary

✓ With exercise comes good pain and bad pain. Good pain is a little muscle soreness that fades away in a couple days. Bad pain is sharp and doesn't go away.

✓ Try the RICE treatment for injuries, and give yourself time to recover. Even better, find out how to prevent injuries altogether.

✓ If you've never had a massage, please book one immediately.

✓ It's okay, even encouraged, to exercise while pregnant. Just take it easy and exercise safely.

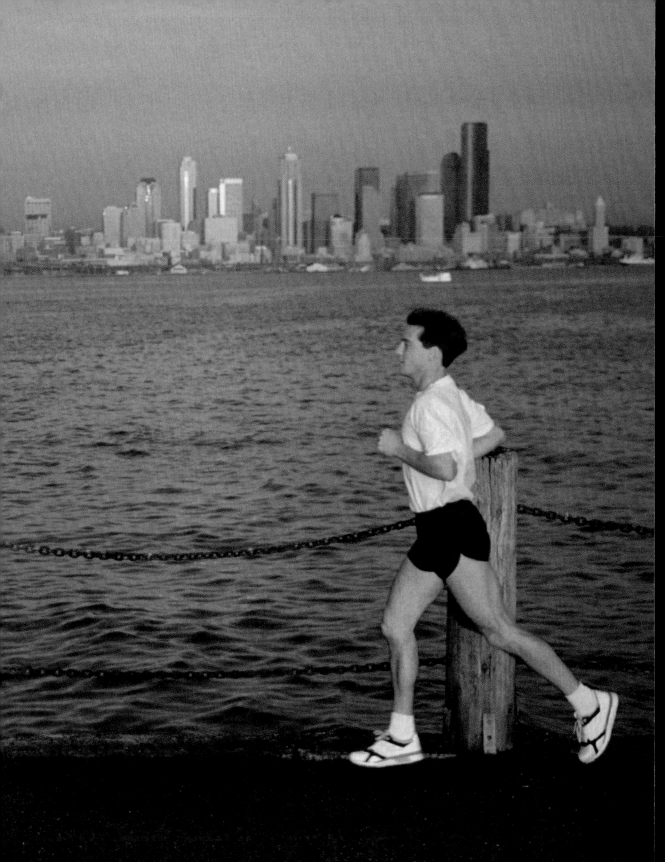

Chapter 17

Exercise for Travellers

WHEN TRAVELLING, you're far from your gym and out of your fitness routine. So are you tempted to throw in the towel and order a rich meal from room service? Don't! There are plenty of ways to stay (or get) fit when you're on the move. Here are a few workout strategies for travellers, including exercises you can do in your hotel room and simple tips to keep you sane on a long flight. If it's a holiday you're planning, why not include physical activity on the itinerary? There are mountains to climb, cities to explore, and country walks to enjoy.

In this chapter...

✓ Be prepared

✓ Hotel room workout strategies

✓ Aeroplane know-how

✓ Altitude adjustment

✓ Fitness adventures

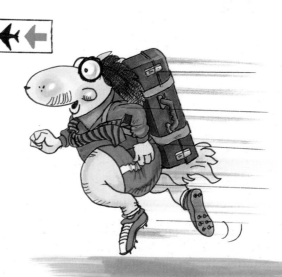

Be prepared

LET'S SAY YOU'VE BEEN FAITHFUL *to your new exercise routine, but you have to go away on business. You'll miss football practice and your morning walk. You're going to be busy all day, and at night you'll probably just collapse in front of the television for a while. After all, it's going to be a long trip, and you're going to be tired.*

Well, if you want to feel great instead of exhausted, prepare for exercise before you go. Call the place you're staying, and find out what facilities they have. Wouldn't you hate it if there was a lovely indoor pool and you forgot your swimming gear?

Many hotels have fitness facilities, so find out what they have before you go so you'll be prepared. Many places without a full-scale gym do at least have small fitness rooms with weights and a treadmill or two.

I love working out in hotel fitness centres because they're nearly always empty. (Perhaps I've just been particularly lucky.) But keep your eye out for shady characters when you're alone in a strange fitness room.

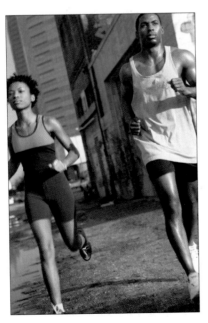

Go exploring

Find out if there's a safe place to run or walk in the area, and bring your running shoes. You'll discover more about the town or city than if you hide out in the hotel room the whole time. Even if you haven't been working out at home, you can still add exercise to your trip. It's reinvigorating and can help you adjust to your new environment.

If you're on a business trip, exercise can make you feel better and subsequently feel better about other people. This can make your trip more successful. People respond better to you if you seem healthy and happy.

■ **One of the best ways** *to get to know the area when you're in a new town or city is on foot – and running is a great way to cover a lot of ground.*

PACKING A FEW ESSENTIALS

What to pack

- Workout clothes for various temperatures (shorts and sweat pants, tank top and sweatshirt, exercise shoes)
- Swimming gear, swim cap, and goggles (if there's a pool; just a costume or trunks if there's a hot tub). Also, bring something you can throw on to walk to the pool
- Plastic barbells that you fill up with water to add weight, or two water bottles
- Your favourite exercise video. If there's a VCR in your room, why not work out to your favourite video?
- Kitchen timer. Why the kitchen timer? As mentioned in Chapter 5, set a kitchen timer for 10, 15, 30 minutes, or whatever you have time for, and turn it on and exercise until the buzzer rings
- Resistance band or tube

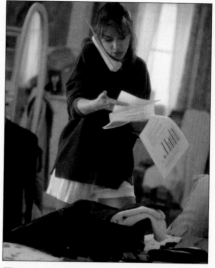

■ **Exercise is a great** *stress buster, so don't go on that important business trip without packing your workout essentials.*

What not to pack

Hauling too much weight around can make your back and neck hurt. These days, people often walk around carrying an entire mobile office. Shed a few pounds. Ask yourself if you really need your laptop on your trip, for example. Many hotels offer business centres where you can check your e-mail. If you decide you do need the laptop, get the lightest one you can, especially if you're going to have to lug it everywhere.

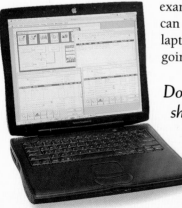

LAPTOP – A WEIGHT TO CARRY

Don't carry all your heavy bags on one shoulder. Try to carry as many bags as you can backpack-style so the weight is evenly distributed on both shoulders. Suitcases with wheels can also relieve you of some extra burden.

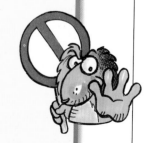

Hotel room workout strategies

THE FITNESS ROOM *is out of order, there's no pool, and it's raining and cold outside. Or, you only have a few minutes, and there's no time to go out for a jog or have a swim in the pool. If this is the case, it's time to institute the hotel room workout strategies.*

Before you go out to meetings, or wherever your travel plans bring you, try a quick cardio blast in the morning to wake you up and get your blood moving. Even if you only have a few minutes, you'll feel alert and ready to face the day. In the evening, if you get in late and don't have a lot of energy, try some gentle stretching to release the stress of the day and get you relaxed for bed.

30-minute full body workout

A little bit of exercise is always better than none, and 30 minutes of exercise is even better.

If you have time for a full workout, either in the morning, in the evening, or smack in the middle of the day, here are some suggestions for a stuck-at-the-hotel 30-minute full body workout.

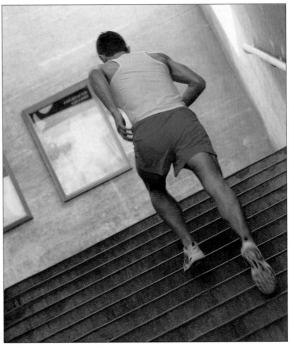

WARM-UP ROUTINE

Warm-up

If the hotel has a well-lit and secure staircase, walk up and down it for 3 minutes, gradually increasing your pace. If you have time, run or walk up and down for 5 more minutes at your top speed. Then, run or walk as fast as possible back to your room, for 1 minute of jumping jacks.

Stretch

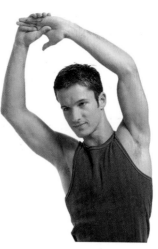

STEP 1

1. Extend both arms overhead, clasp your hands, and stretch back as far as you can. Open up your chest and breathe. Hold the above position, then bend your knees slightly and stretch to each side as far as you can

2. Squat down as far as you can, put your hands on the floor, and gently straighten your legs

3. Lie on your back on the floor and cross your left ankle above your right knee, left knee out to the side. Place both hands behind your right thigh and pull toward your chest. Switch sides

4. Pull both knees to your chest, and rotate both knees to the left, and breathe deeply. Switch sides

5. Lie on your stomach, and put both hands under each shoulder, and straighten your arms as far as you can until you feel a stretch in your lower back

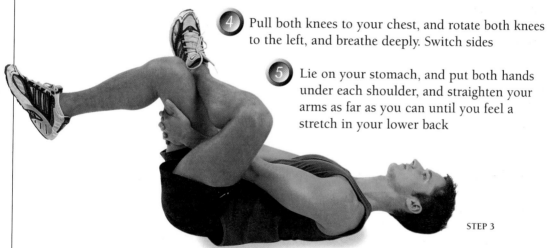

STEP 3

Strength training

Try a round of these exercises (descriptions in Part 3). Do two or three sets of the suggested reps or as many as you can, and go directly to the next exercise.

1. 10–15 push-ups

2. 10–15 squats

3. 10 lunges (each side)

4. 20 crunches

To finish off your hotel workout, repeat the stretches above.

Resistance band workout

A resistance band (this was introduced in Chapter 5) is a great travel workout aid because it's an effective resistance-training tool and yet it folds up into the tiniest of spaces. There are different brands and styles, but basically a resistance band looks like a giant rubber band (some have handles), and you stretch it to work your muscles.

For these exercises, you need a resistance band or tube with handles, one that's long enough for you to stretch from the floor to over your head. They come in different levels of resistance – try a pliable tube to start off with.

Work up to 20 reps, and move on to the next exercise.

Work up to 20 reps with your resistance band workout. If it's your first time, start with five or however many you can or have time to do.

Do all the following exercises in order, without resting in between, to get an added cardio workout.

Squat press

This works your thighs (quads), backs of legs (hamstrings), shoulders (deltoids), and the backs of your arms (triceps).

1. Start by standing on the tube with your feet hip-width apart and arms by your sides, palms up, holding the ends of the tube. With your shoulders back, and chest forward, inhale and squat back as if you were sitting in a chair. As you sit, bend your arms so that your hands are in front of your shoulders. Elbows should be right above knees. Make sure that your knees are over your feet and not extended over your toes during the squat

2. Next, exhale and rise, straightening your arms over your head, while turning your palms forward. When your arms are straight, squeeze your shoulders, contracting the muscles

3. Slowly lower your arms while turning your palms so they face behind you, working the triceps as you bring your arms down as before, and squat again

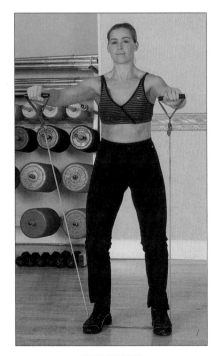

SQUAT PRESS

One-arm chest lift

Works the chest (pectorals) and front shoulder muscles (deltoids).

Start by standing with your feet on the tube, hip-width apart. With a straight back, abs tight, and shoulders back, place one hand on your hip and one straight by your side, while holding the band. Exhale and extend the straight arm up and across your body, keeping your elbow straight but not locked. Contract your chest muscles at the top. Lower slowly and repeat for desired reps, then repeat with the other arm.

Upright row

Works the front and side shoulder muscles (deltoids).

1 Once again, stand with your feet on the tube, hip-width apart. Keep your back straight (not arched), shoulders back, and chest out. Pull the tube straight up to your shoulders, palms in, with your elbows out. Keep the tube in line with your legs and body. At the top of the movement, your hands should be in front of your shoulders, and elbows out at shoulder height. Lower to starting position

2 Raise the tube again, this time out to the side with your arms straight but not locked, until your arms are straight out to the sides at shoulder height. Lower to starting position, and repeat for desired reps

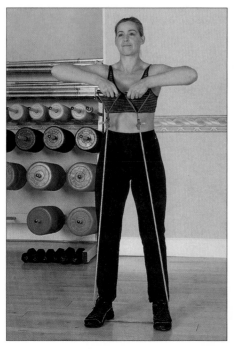

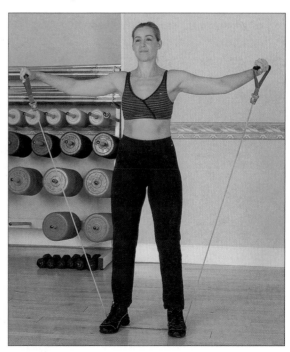

UPRIGHT ROW 1   UPRIGHT ROW 2

Overhead press

Works the backs of arms (triceps) and shoulders (deltoids).

Stand with your back straight, and one foot behind you standing on the tube. With both hands, raise the tube straight overhead, then slowly lower behind your head. Your elbows should be up by your temples, hands behind head. Lift the tube back up so your arms are straight but not locked. Repeat for desired reps.

Forward curl

Works the upper arms (biceps).

Stand with your feet on the tube, hip-width apart. With your back straight, shoulders back and arms by your sides, and with palms up, curl your arms up as in a basic bicep curl. Lower slowly and repeat for desired reps.

Side curl

Works the upper arms (biceps).

The position is the same as the forward curl above, but turn palms out and bend the arms up away from the body. At the top, your palms should face your body, at shoulder height. Lower and repeat.

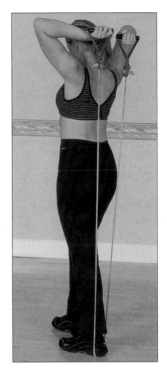

OVERHEAD PRESS

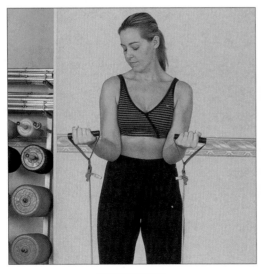

FORWARD CURL

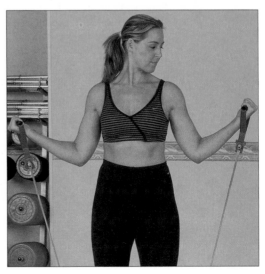

SIDE CURL

Aeroplane know-how

FLYING CAN TAKE A LOT OUT OF YOU. Instead of arriving exhausted, try these simple tips to keep you feeling good while you fly.

Drink up

If you've ever flown, you know this already: the air in the cabin of an aeroplane is extremely dry. That's why it's extra important to stay hydrated. Try to drink quarter of a litre of water (8 oz) for every hour you're on the plane, and avoid dehydrating liquid like coffee and alcohol. If you must have those, order a water chaser.

Get up

Get out of your seat and walk around whenever you can, especially on a long flight. Roam the aisle, or stand at the back of the plane (the cabin crew really love this). If the drinks trolley is in your way or the seat belt sign is on, then stretch in your seat. Stretch your arms out in front of you, bend and arch your back, roll your head and shoulders, and rotate your ankles.

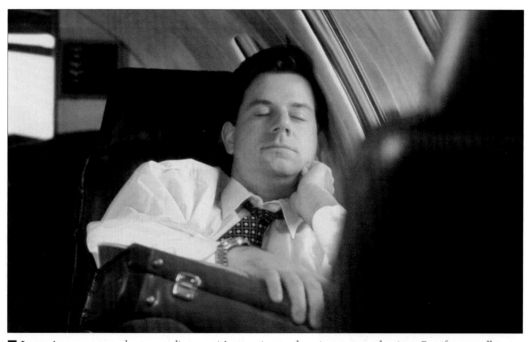

■ **Long journeys** *can be very tedious, so it's tempting to sleep just to pass the time. But if you really want to arrive feeling fresh, be sure to get up, move around, and stretch every so often.*

A good in-flight neck stretch

Reach over your head with your left arm, and gently put your hand on the right side of your head. Lean your head to the left, and gently pull your head over with your hand for an extra stretch. Keep your shoulders down and relaxed, and take a deep breath. Switch to the other side.

Breathe

Take a deep, relaxing yoga breath. Sit up straight, but relaxed. Let your hands relax by your sides. Inhale slowly, filling your lower belly, upper belly, and chest with air. Then, slowly exhale, emptying your chest, then your belly of air. On the exhale, concentrate on pulling your belly back towards your spine. Then repeat.

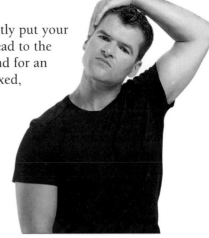

■ **This neck stretch** *and other exercises can be done in your seat to help prevent stiffness brought on by a long flight.*

Avoid jet lag

Flying to another time zone takes a toll on your body. It upsets your circadian rhythm, which is your internal clock that tells you when to sleep, wake up, and eat. This can give you a headache, make you feel dizzy, and upset your stomach. To lessen the effects of zinging to another time zone, as soon as you get on the plane, change your watch to the time of your destination.

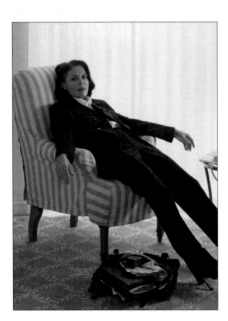

Try to sleep when it's night there. You could try a sleep aid, or have a glass of red wine (and water). Also, eat at the mealtime of your destination, even if that means bringing your own snack on the plane. These little changes will help you adjust to the new time zone a bit faster.

■ **Jet lag** *can be very debilitating – but by making little changes you can help your body clock adapt to a new routine more quickly.*

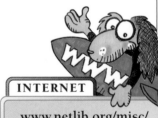

INTERNET

www.netlib.org/misc/
jet-lag-diet

If you're feeling ambitious, this web site has a feast, fast, feast diet that is supposed to keep you in top shape while traveling to different time zones. The plan is a little hard to follow, but if jet lag is a problem for you, check it out.

Altitude adjustment

IF YOU LIVE AT SEA LEVEL and travel to a high altitude, you're going to feel a difference. Any altitude over 2,600 metres (8,000 feet) can have a noticeable effect on your body. The reason for this is that when you're this high you take in less oxygen with every breath. This can cause mild to extreme symptoms. Most people experience mild altitude sickness like headache, nausea, and weakness. It can happen to anyone, regardless of age, sex, or size. For some reason, on some trips to the mountains I get sick, and on others I feel fine. The same person may not know what to expect from trip to trip.

What can you do to avoid feeling sick? Be aware that you're not going to be able to do as much physical activity as usual without getting winded. You have to take more breaths to get the oxygen you're used to, so you get winded easily.

Avoid overexerting yourself on the first day or two at a high altitude. Also, drink lots of water, and avoid salt and heavy foods. Alcohol at a higher elevation can feel twice as strong; one drink up there can feel like two at sea level. Drink lots of extra water, and take an ibuprofen to stave off altitude sickness.

The best way to avoid altitude sickness is to acclimatize, which means going up to a higher elevation gradually. It takes about 1–3 days to acclimatize to a new altitude. Given time, your body can adjust to the decrease in oxygen.

When you acclimatize, your body adjusts to operating on less oxygen by increasing the depth of respiration and by producing more red blood cells to carry the oxygen.

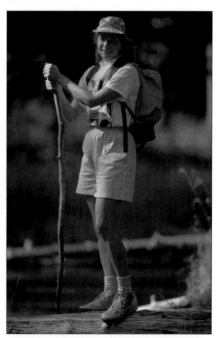

■ **When walking** *at high altitude, don't push yourself too hard – it's important to give your body time to acclimatize.*

Fitness adventures

*WHILE BUSINESS TRAVEL usually means trying to squeeze in a hotel
room workout when you can, travelling on holiday is another story. Exercise
and adventure should be on the itinerary for a fun break.*

A holiday centred on physical activity can kick off a fitness programme and provide
you with a goal to work towards. For example, you'll be better able to take advantage
of a trip to the mountains if you're in good shape to enjoy the great outdoors. Also,
many a trip to a warm climate in the dead of winter has prompted a mad dash to get
a bikini-ready body. Although looking great on the beach is certainly a perk, a more
inspiring goal comes from the inside; get in better shape so you can enjoy yourself.
A nice-looking body is a welcome by-product.

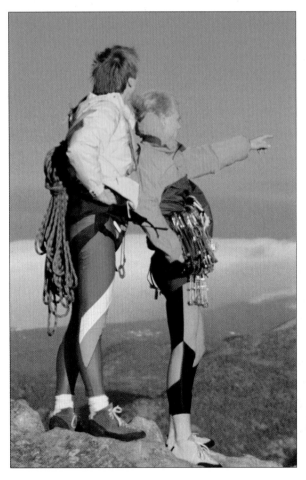

Fit in some fun

Getting ready for a trip that's a few
months, or weeks (or days) away is
a great workout goal. But, if there's
no time to prepare, don't worry.
You can get physical when you get
there. You might even be inspired
to continue exercising when you
come home. An adventure-oriented
trip with family or friends, alone,
or with a group can be fun. You'll
be too busy having fun to think
about getting exercise or staying
fit, you'll just be doing it.

There are adventures, fitness retreats,
and spas calling your name. There is
something for everyone. A short list
follows to give you an idea of what's
out there. Try something you've
never done before.

■ **Trying a new activity** *can prove to
be a real voyage of discovery. Challenge
yourself to do something different as a
way of getting fit.*

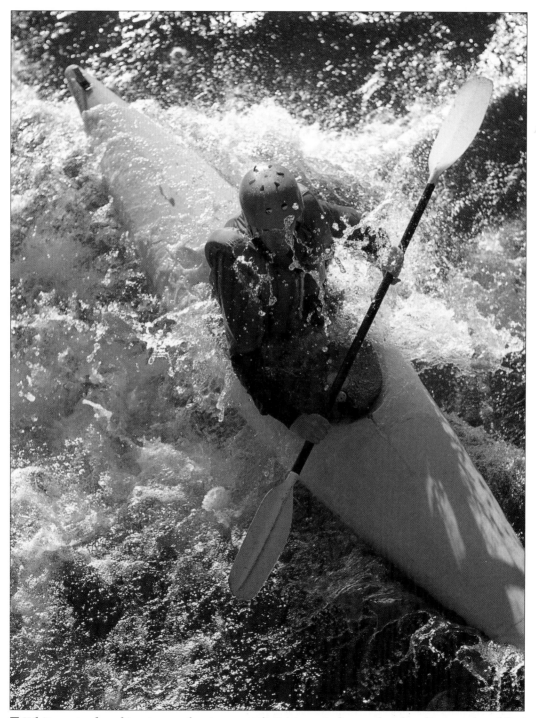

■ **White water kayaking** *is one adventure sport that's guaranteed to get the adrenaline pumping while the upper body gets a rigorous physical workout.*

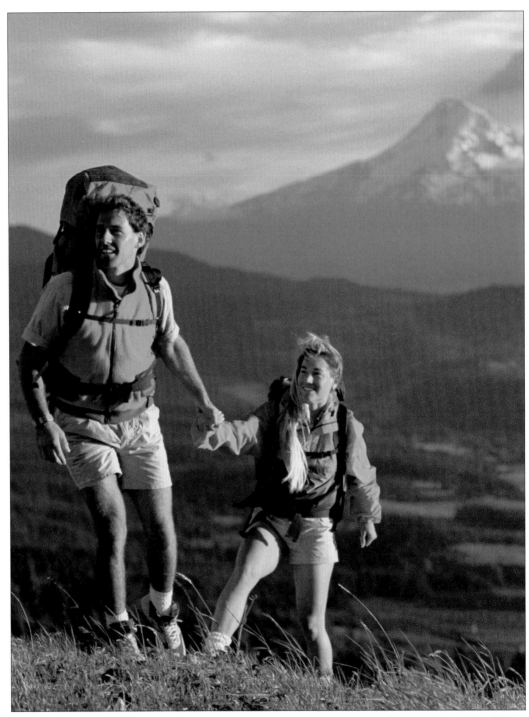

■ **There are many different walking tours** *to choose from, so shop around for one that will enable you to experience the kind of scenery you find uplifting and that suits your ability and pocket.*

Walking, hiking, or biking tours

Options for these tours run the gamut from a walking tour that consists of an afternoon of leisurely sightseeing, to a 2-week-long hiking trip in rugged terrain. These tours are a great way to explore a foreign country, new city, or terrain you've never seen or experienced before. There are tours for every skill level, whether you want to stroll around cities or cycle 20 miles a day. These tours are usually done in groups, and depending on the package, they often include meals and accommodation, and a guide who leads you to some spectacular destinations. Imagine waking up and instead of thinking, "I have to get in a 60-minute walk today", thinking, "I can't wait to explore the Irish countryside today!" There are multi-city and single-city tours, rural or urban settings. For some of them you camp out at night, others put you up in a luxury hotel or, perhaps, in a quaint countryside inn.

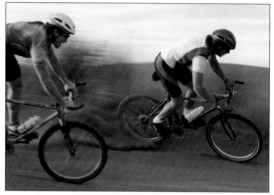

■ **If you're interested in exploring** *picturesque countryside, why not tour by bike? You'll have the freedom of the open road, plus the option of setting your own pace.*

Things to consider

Price range: this can vary considerably.

What's included: find out what's included and what's going to cost extra. If it's a bike tour, find out how much it will cost to rent a bike, for example.

Duration: how long can you go for? Some last a few days; others last several weeks. Some walking tours might even last only a few hours.

Group dynamic: most have group-size limits. Find out what they are. Do you want a large group to socialize with or a more intimate setting? Also find out who goes on the particular trip. Some trips are more family-orientated, others are just for men or women, gay, straight, single, in couples, older, or younger. Of course, most of the groups will be a mixed bag, but some cater more to certain demographics.

Level of fitness: find out what you'll be expected to do on a daily basis. Most tours can accommodate various fitness levels, but some are definitely more challenging than others. Find the one that suits your current level of fitness best, so you can be challenged, but not struggling.

Location: want to explore the busy streets and sights of Paris or hike through fields of wildflowers where it seems that no other human has trod? Some tours provide urban and rural settings while some specialize in one or the other. Find out before you go.

THE LOWDOWN ON SPAS

People once went to spas primarily for health concerns. Many certainly still do that, but spas have become very popular over the past few years not only as places to get healthy but also as places to be pampered and spoiled rotten. Spas are not just for women; many men frequent spas these days. Here's a simple rundown of the different kinds of spas:

Spa retreat

This is a place where every activity and amenity is oriented toward mind-body-spirit wellbeing. These retreats are private places in beautiful settings where guests often stay the same length of time to share the experience of total renewal.

> **DEFINITION**
>
> **Spa cuisine** *is healthy food that is low in fat and calories.*

They feature a wide array of indoor and outdoor fitness options, healthy *spa cuisine*, relaxing treatments, and educational and inspirational programs. A stay at a spa retreat is a good way to get back in touch with yourself, if you've had a life change, or just need some "me-time".

Luxury spa retreat

This is an intimate, elegant spa where a small number of guests (often all women) are pampered by an attentive staff. These have a serene ambiance and often feature gourmet spa cuisine and individualized beauty, fitness, and wellness programmes. This is the spoiled rotten scenario.

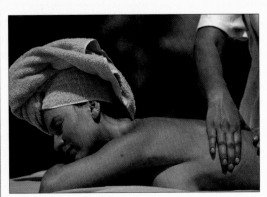

■ **Most spas** *offer a wide range of beauty and body treatments, such as massage.*

Resort spa

This is a good one to go to if you'd like to add some golf, tennis, or swimming to your spa experience. Here you'll find all the resort amenities with spa services as well. Spa cuisine is usually offered along with traditional fare and alcohol. This is a good choice if you're travelling with your family, or with someone who wants to participate in non-spa activities. There are also luxury resort spas, which are similar except they're usually a bit more secluded, and, well, expensive.

Weight management spa

This type of spa is designed to help you lose weight. It specializes in lifestyle changes, rather than the quick fix. Weight management spas are usually medically orientated with physician supervision.

Wellness retreat

This is a facility that addresses each guest's specific health issues. It's a good option if you have health problems, or if you're interested in learning how to live a healthier life. Some retreats are traditionally medical; others take a more holistic approach.

Holistic retreat

Unlike the luxury spa retreat, the holistic retreat is generally unadorned, and located in a rustic environment. These places often specialize in yoga and meditation, and offer vegetarian cuisine. Many offer hiking and massage. They all strive to unite the mind, body, and spirit.

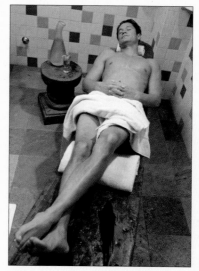

■ **Even if you don't want** *to stay at a spa, you can still enjoy being pampered. Day spas offer treatments by appointment, so you can visit whenever you feel in need of rejuvenation.*

Adventure spa

This is for the physically fit spa goer who wants an exciting, challenging experience in the outdoors. These spas are often located in dramatic wilderness settings and offer hiking, climbing, horseback riding, and other outdoor fun.

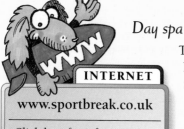

INTERNET

www.sportbreak.co.uk

Click here for information on spa and activity holidays throughout the UK.

Day spa

This is a local spa that you go to for specific treatments. Instead of staying overnight, you call and schedule a massage, facial, or other spa treatment.

Plan your own adventure

Of course you can always plan your own adventure, or maybe weave a little extra activity into an already-planned trip. Take a trip to the mountains in the winter where you can downhill or cross-country ski, hike, snowshoe, and explore. Cross-country skiing is a fabulous full-body cardio workout and is great because you don't have to worry about tumbling down a mountain. Don't know how to ski? No problem; take a lesson. Break out of your comfort zone, and try something new.

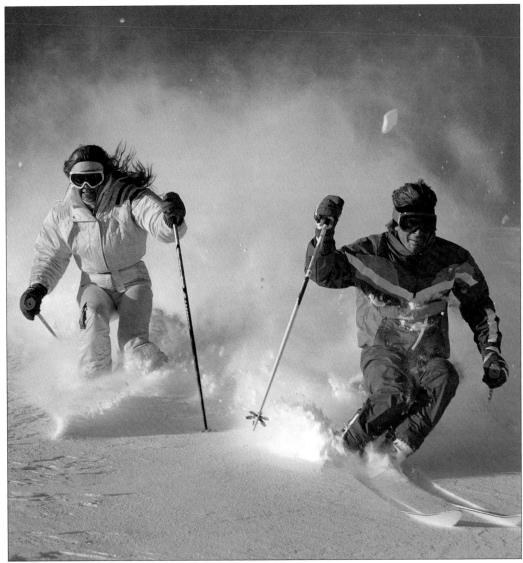

■ **Skiing works out the whole body** *as well as being an invigorating and fun way to explore the mountainside. If you're a novice, take a few lessons and see how you fare on the piste.*

I used to hate skiing. All my friends were much better than I was, and they looked great in their ski clothes while I left shameful blue prints down the slope with my soggy jeans. On a recent trip to the mountains, though, I had a long, private ski lesson, and suddenly everything clicked. I got over my fear of the mountain and wanted to ski more!

Ski resorts are fun in the summer, too. You can hike and mountain bike on trails covered in beautiful wildflowers, swim in a lake, or frolic in the grass. Try your hand at rock climbing. Or if it's a beach trip you're after, instead of sitting under the umbrella all day, jump into the ocean, build a sandcastle, or take a long stroll down the beach.

The best thing about going on an adventure is that it can change your outlook. It might inspire you to go on local adventures when you get home. There is a lovely park near my house that I sometimes forget about, but whenever I return from some outside adventure, I get home and hit the park with renewed vigour. Check it out for yourself – explore, have fun, get fit!

A simple summary

✔ Find out what fitness options you'll have when you're going on a trip, so you can pack accordingly and take advantage of them.

✔ Just because you're stuck in your hotel room on a business trip doesn't mean you have to miss your workout. Try some simple hotel room exercises.

✔ Arrive happy. Flying can take a lot out of you, but you can stay on top by drinking water, stretching, and adjusting your inner clock quickly when your travels take you across time zones.

✔ High altitudes means less oxygen, which means you'll get winded faster. Drink water, ascend slowly, and take it easy on the first day at a high altitude to keep sickness at bay.

✔ There are fitness adventures for every taste. Take a walking tour, climb a mountain, or get pampered at a spa.

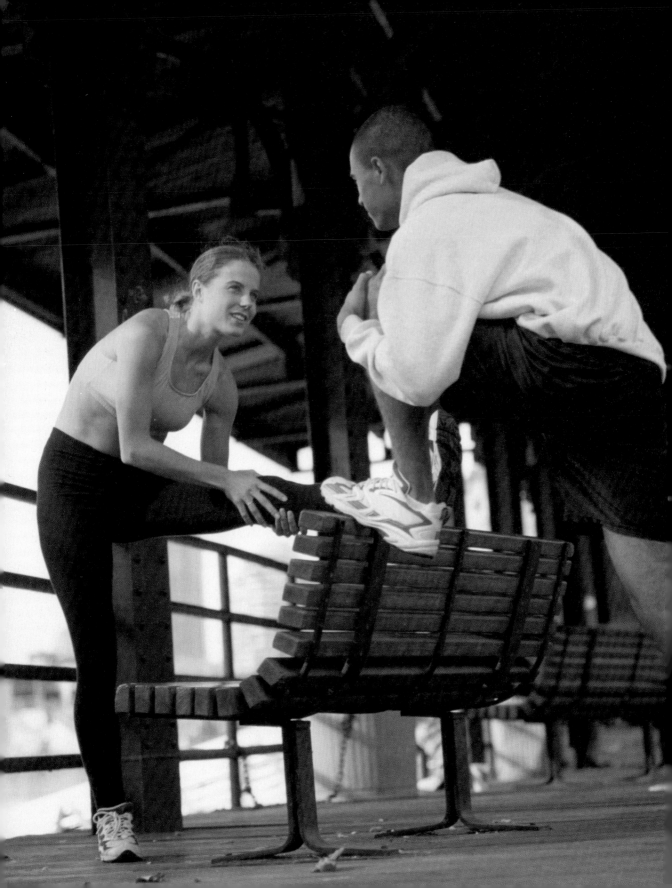

Chapter 18

Keep It Fun

I F YOU'VE BEEN EXERCISING FAITHFULLY for months but you feel as if you're not making any progress, don't get discouraged. Now is the time to take a look at how far you've come since you started and reassess your goals. When it's time to bring your exercise routine to the next level, there are plenty of ways to increase the intensity, duration, and frequency. We'll take a look at some tricks professional athletes use to keep their fitness routines fresh and challenging. And you'll find out how to tell if your exercise routine is doing more harm than good.

In this chapter...

✓ Hitting a plateau

✓ Get to the next level

✓ Variety is the spice of life

✓ Simple ways to revamp your routine

✓ Give me a break

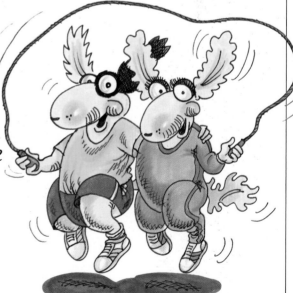

IF YOU USUALLY EXERCISE ALONE, SCHEDULE A SESSION OR TWO WITH A FRIEND TO VARY THE ROUTINE

Hitting a plateau

PEOPLE WHO DROP OUT *of fitness programmes often do so because they have hit a plateau and don't know how to get over it. This usually happens within the first 6 months. They get frustrated that progress is so slow, and they quit. Of the people who make it through those crucial months, half do just enough to stay fit, but not enough to see results.*

Time for a rethink

If you've been exercising faithfully but lately it feels as if you're not making any gains, maybe you too have hit a plateau. If your routine – whether it's lifting weights, running on the treadmill, or a combination of exercises – starts to feel easy, you're ready to revamp it. When you hit a plateau, the weight you've been lifting doesn't make your muscles sore any more, and it's harder to get to your target heart rate when you exercise aerobically. As your heart gets stronger, it's harder to raise your heart rate. (This is a good thing.)

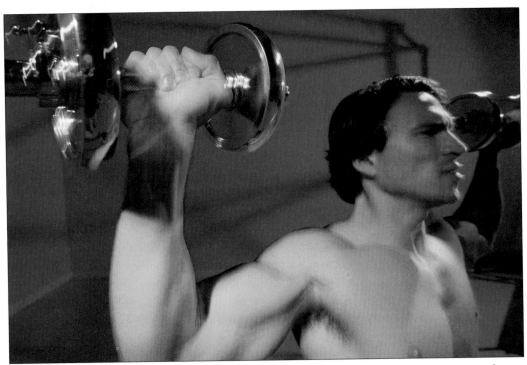

■ **If you're able to complete** *your workout with minimal effort, it's time to adjust your routine. If you don't keep pushing yourself, you won't see any improvement and may end up feeling discouraged.*

Get to the next level

WHEN YOUR ROUTINE BECOMES STALE and you're not getting results, it's time to make some changes. The best way to assess and mend your situation is by keeping an exercise diary and taking a look at your current goals. This helps you see how you can keep your fitness routine productive, and also keep it interesting and fresh.

Remember those fitness diaries?

One way to get over this bump in the road to fitness is to take a look at your fitness diary. If you haven't been keeping one, now is a great time to start.

People who keep fitness diaries tend to make faster progress in their programmes, are more satisfied with their progress, and stay with their routines for longer than people who don't record their workouts. When you can't see your progress, you might feel frustrated and want to quit.

After every workout, write in your diary; include the exercises completed and how you felt during the workout. Refer to this to keep track of your progress, and to determine what changes need to be made to your programme.

Gauge your results by comparing today's performance against last week's. Maybe you've been doing the same workout, but it's easier now. That means you're getting in better shape, whether you realize it or not.

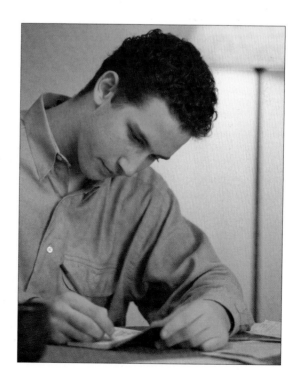

■ **Record each workout** *and describe how you feel as you're doing it. It's very satisfying to look over a fitness diary and see how much progress you've made.*

Remember how far you've come

Instead of lamenting the fact that you don't seem to be making gains as fast as you want or as quickly as you did when you first started, look back at the beginning. You're probably a lot better off than you were before you started exercising.

Congratulate yourself on what you've done so far, and move on.

Reassess your goals

If you're ready to get to the next level but you're feeling stuck, maybe it's time to reassess your goals. In general, your long-term goals should be beyond your current abilities, but not so far off that you get discouraged. Rethink your long-term goals; are they realistic? If you haven't done so already, break down your long-term goals into smaller, more attainable short-term goals.

Be flexible and allow yourself to adjust your goals if you need to. If your original goal was to lose 5 kilos, but it seems to be taking forever and you just want to skip the aerobics class and eat cake, then break that goal down into bite-sized pieces.

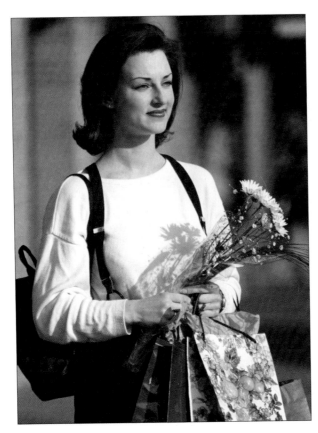

Start with a goal of losing 2 kilos (5 lbs). When you reach that goal, buy yourself a new CD (or some other small reward). Then, set a new goal of losing another 2–3 kilos (5-7 lbs). People make the best progress when they successfully work towards a series of short-term goals, and are rewarded at frequent intervals.

Frequent rewards give you a feeling of accomplishment and encourage you to forge ahead.

■ **Buy yourself** *a small present, such as a CD, book, or a bunch of flowers, as a way of patting yourself on the back each time you achieve a short-term goal.*

Variety is the spice of life

IF YOU'VE BEEN DOING THE SAME THING for 3 days a week for a year, you'll maintain your current level of fitness, but you won't improve. In order to make progress, you should change your exercises every few weeks. Change your workout in little ways every couple of weeks, and change your routine dramatically three or four times a year.

Ideally, you'll always have a few different workouts in rotation. Varying your workout is the best way to combat boredom, burnout, and injury. If you exercise every day, alternating exercises allows muscles time to recover, prevents injuries, and promotes a higher level of fitness.

Change your routine

Improvement comes from stressing the muscles and allowing them to recover, not from doing exactly the same workout every day. You can exercise your heart with aerobic exercise every day, but skeletal muscles start to break down when exercised intensely more than a few times a week. And besides, doing the same workout day in, day out can put a damper on motivation. Fortunately, there are plenty of ways to mix it up.

Changing your routine will keep you physically and mentally challenged and entertained. To improve fitness, you need to increase the duration, intensity, and frequency of your workouts. Easier said than done? Take a look at some of the methods that we've borrowed from professional athletes to create new challenges.

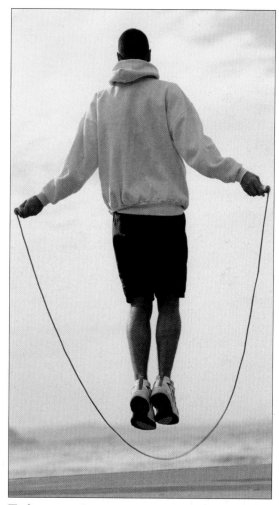

■ **If you enjoy skipping,** *why not incorporate it into your fitness routine? You're more likely to exercise if you keep yourself entertained.*

Simple ways to revamp your routine

SINCE PROFESSIONAL ATHLETES *are constantly training, it's important for them to mix it up and keep their workouts interesting and productive. You can adapt some of their tricks for your own fitness routines, whatever your goals. Try cross training, interval training, the hard–easy principle, circuit training, and supersets, and you'll be exercising like a pro.*

Trivia...

Marathon runners are injured more frequently than triathletes, who compete in three sports. Even though triathletes exercise more, they exercise different muscle groups on successive days. They run one day and swim or cycle the next.

Cross training

In cross training you engage in two or more types of exercises either in one workout or in successive workouts. For example, you might play football one day and swim laps the next. The great thing about cross training is that it keeps the workouts interesting, develops your entire body, and distributes the training load among different body parts. This reduces the risk of injury.

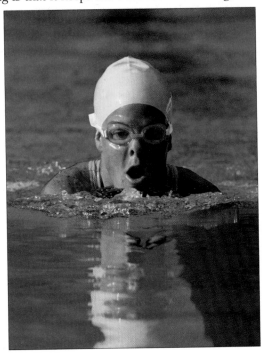

Running 30 minutes a day and riding a bike 30 minutes the next day is far less likely to cause injury than if you did both every day for 15 minutes.

Cross training allows you to continue training when you're injured, as long as you avoid using the injured area. If you sprain your wrist, you can still take a long walk.

■ **Swimming is a good activity** *to alternate with more demanding aerobic exercise, such as jogging or running, because it doesn't stress the muscles or joints in the same way.*

Follow the pros

Professional athletes employ cross training all the time so that they don't do the same exercises every day. For example, a distance runner in training might lift weights twice a week, stretch every day, and bike once a week in addition to her running regimen.

Of course it's not just for the pros: fitness enthusiasts cross train all the time. If you've been hitting the gym for weight training and playing on a hockey team, for example, then you're already cross training. Any good fitness routine is going to use cross training to some degree because stretching, strength training, and aerobic exercise are all basic components of a well-rounded programme.

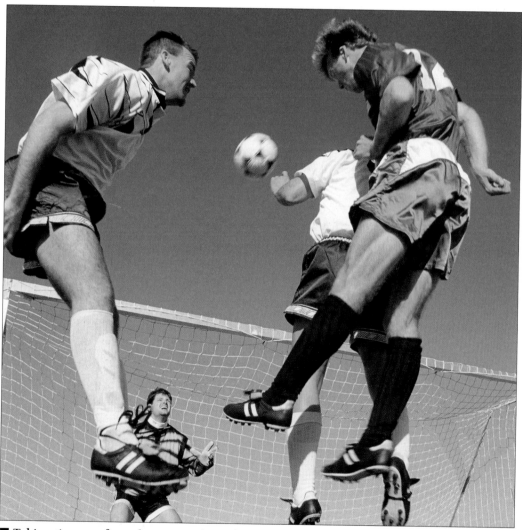

■ **Taking time out from the gym** *to play a game of football two or three times a week helps reduce the risk of injury. This is because a varied routine exerts different muscle groups.*

CROSS-TRAINING PROGRAMME

This 1-week programme is good for all-around conditioning. It can help boost aerobic fitness, muscle strength, muscle endurance, and flexibility, and can also help you shed a few kilos by burning a fair number of calories each day.

Day of the week	Activity	Minutes
Monday	● Brisk walk with hand weights ● Stretch ● Upper body weight training	30 10 20
Tuesday	● Light jog ● Stretch ● Lower body weight training	20 10 30
Wednesday	● Swimming ● Yoga	20 30
Thursday	● Cycling, rowing, or cross-country skiing (either the real thing or exercise machine) ● Stretch	 30 15
Friday	● Brisk walk ● Upper and lower body weight training	20 30
Saturday	● Jog ● Stretch	30 15
Sunday	● Leisurely stroll	30

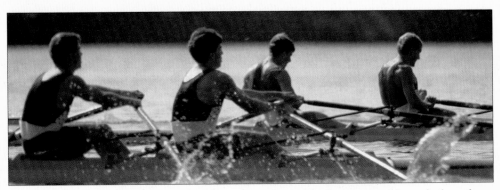

■ **Rowing is an excellent form** *of aerobic exercise that works the upper and lower body at the same time, making it an ideal activity to include in a cross-training programme.*

Interval training

Another thing to have in your bag of workout tricks is interval training, which is a method of varying the intensity of your workout session. Interval training entails alternating short bursts of intense activity with a less intense form of exercise. The secret to interval training is to exercise beyond your comfort level, but only in brief spurts. You can interval train with any aerobic exercise. You go all out for a minute, then you return to your normal pace. Then you go all out again at a high level of intensity, and return to your normal pace again. Interval training helps build muscle rapidly. Mix it in once or twice a week with your regular exercise, and you'll leap over that exercise plateau.

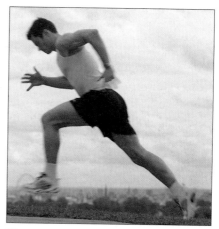

■ **A runner** *would interval train by alternating brief spurts of speed with periods of running at a normal pace.*

When you start out, your interval to rest ratio should be about 1:3, so if you run fast for 20 seconds, walk for 1 minute. As you improve, decrease your recovery periods slowly so that your interval and recovery times are the same. You should also increase your intensity and the number of short bursts you do as you get better.

Interval training is a way to increase the intensity of your workout, burn more calories, and inject spice into a stale routine. It helps build and preserve muscle tone and promote cardiovascular health.

TYPICAL INTERVAL WORKOUT

This interval workout can be incorporated into your routine a couple of times a week to improve muscle tone and cardiovascular health.

1. Warm-up for 20 minutes with a brisk walk or light jog

2. Run as fast as you can for 20 seconds

3. Slow down and jog lightly or walk for 1 minute

4. Repeat steps 2 and 3 with the aim of doing four to six quick sprints

Increase the pace

An easy way to incorporate interval training into your workout is by spontaneously revving up the speed in whatever you're doing. If you're on a walk, walk for a while at a regular pace, then walk as fast as you can for a minute or two, then walk slowly again. You can play games like running as fast as you can to a certain tree or lamppost, then walk for a few minutes and do it again. This type of exercise is sometimes called fartlek training.

Fartlek training (fartlek is a Swedish word that means "speed play") is a kind of interval training. Unlike regular interval training, fartlek training doesn't involve accurately measured intervals. Instead, how you feel determines the length and speed of each interval.

I like fartlek training because I'd rather listen to my body instead of keeping my eye on a watch. I think it's more fun to suddenly sprint until I don't feel like sprinting any more, then jog lightly until the next spontaneous outburst.

The hard–easy principle

The hard–easy principle is a standard training method that was created by a long-distance-running coach. It's a method that is often used by runners, but can be applied to any exercise programme. The hard–easy principle dictates that in order to attain higher levels of fitness, a person should exercise intensely two or three times a week, and less intensely on the other days. So it's two or three hard workouts separated by easier recovery days. This is based on the same theory that requires 48 hours between exercising muscle groups to give them time to recover.

> **DEFINITION**
>
> *To **overload** means to do a harder-than-average workout. With cardio, that means to make it more intense; with weight training it means to add more weight than usual. **Underload** is an easier-than-average workout.*

On the hard days, the exerciser should *overload* and on the easy days, *underload*. On the hard days, you should exercise long and hard enough to cause muscle ache. This will build speed and endurance. Follow that with an easy day where you don't push yourself.

Varying your effort

This training method provides variety, relaxation, and focus. You know you can relax on the easy days and focus all your energy on the hard days. Competitive athletes often need to sports-specific train every day. That is, a professional basketball player will play basketball every day.

To avoid injuries, a basketball player might employ the hard–easy principle by playing a long practice game one day, followed by an easy practice day of going over plays and shooting. In this way, the hard workouts cause less muscle damage.

An easy day isn't for resting, it's just for a less intense workout. For example, an easy day for a marathon runner might be to run 40 kilometres at a relaxed pace.

You can incorporate the hard–easy principle into any fitness routine. For example, you could sign up for an intense class like cardio kickboxing that meets 2 days a week, and on the other days, take a long walk, brisk jog, or swim.

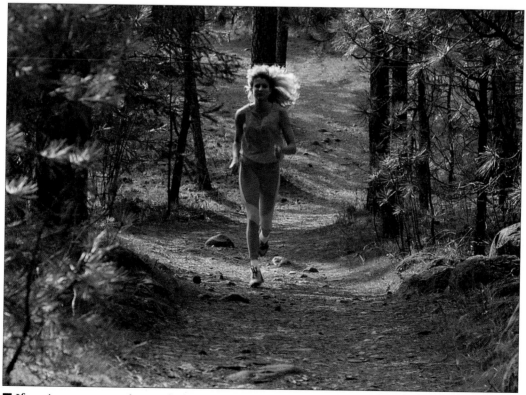

■ **If you're a runner,** *adopting the hard–easy principle would involve running at maximum intensity one day, followed by a more relaxed jog the next day.*

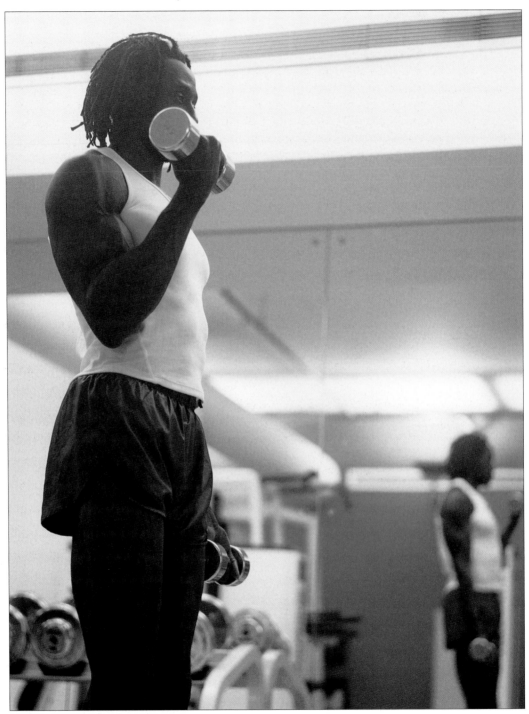

■ **To circuit train in a gym,** *you need to plan carefully. It's important that you don't pause for too long between exercises, so you may have to visit at a quiet time to ensure access to all the equipment you need.*

Circuit training

Circuit training is an excellent way to simultaneously improve mobility and build strength and stamina. The circuit-training format uses a group of six to ten exercises that are completed one right after the other. Each exercise is performed for a specified number of repetitions or for a prescribed time period before moving on to the next exercise. The exercises within each circuit are separated by little or no rest intervals, and each circuit is separated from the next by a longer rest period. The total number of circuits performed during a training session may vary from two to six depending on your level of fitness and energy.

To put together your own circuit workout, think about the possible exercises that can be performed with the available equipment. This will vary depending on where you'll be – the gym, the track, or even at home.

INTERNET

www.primusweb.com/
fitnesspartner/library/
activity/garden

This web site has a fun article on how to "circuit train" in your garden, using exercises like pulling weeds and shovelling.

Try to choose exercises that work each muscle group.

Once you've decided on six or more exercises, write them in the order you want to do them, and note how long it should take to do each one. When you're ready to exercise, put your list somewhere you can see it. Complete all the exercises with little or no rest between, and when you're done, *voilà*, that's one circuit. Try to do two to six circuits with a short rest between. As you improve, you can increase the time for each exercise, and shorten the rest period between the exercises and between the circuits.

■ **Squats are good exercises** *to include in a circuit training routine because they work many of the lower body muscles – and there's no equipment needed.*

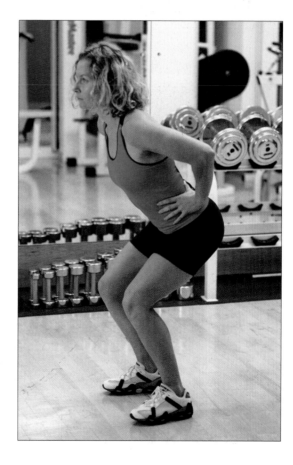

CIRCUIT TRAINING WORKOUT

Here's a sample circuit training workout you can do at home. Before you try it, look over the entire list and make sure you have room to do all the exercises, because the idea is that you don't stop between the exercises. You'll need enough room on the floor for push-ups and crunches and a chair for the tricep dips. If you don't have a raised platform for the calf raises, just do them without one.

Repeat each exercise for 45 seconds, with 15 seconds in between to transition to the next. Instead of counting how many push-ups you do, for example, do however many you can for 45 seconds, and move on to crunches. Remember that the timing may vary depending on your fitness level, and you can adjust it as needed.

Another way to perform this circuit workout is to count reps instead of seconds. Begin with a warm-up by jogging in place for 5 minutes, stretch, perform the workout, then cool down and stretch. For detailed descriptions on how to do each exercise, see Part Three.

1 **Squats** (45 seconds)
15-second rest

2 **Push-ups** (45 seconds)
15-second rest

3 **Crunches** (45 seconds)
15-second rest

4 **Calf raises** (45 seconds)
15-second rest

5 **Triceps dips** (45 seconds)
15-second rest

6 **Alternating lunges** (45 seconds)
15-second rest

7 **Leg extensions** (45 seconds)
Repeat for 2 or 3 cycles.

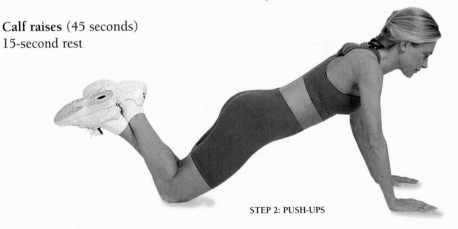

STEP 2: PUSH-UPS

Supersets

A superset is a method that is used primarily for strength training. In the superset method you do two or more exercises in a row, then rest. Normally, if you were to perform three sets of biceps curls, for example, you would rest before moving on to the next exercise. In a superset, after your set of biceps curls you go to the next exercise without stopping.

When you're doing two exercises in a row, it's important to train opposing muscle groups. Some exercises that go together in a superset are biceps curls and triceps dips, overhead press and chest press, or leg extensions and single leg curls.

Although this method condenses exercise time and builds muscle quickly, don't try it until you're already comfortable with the weights or weight machines. Then slowly work these into your routine.

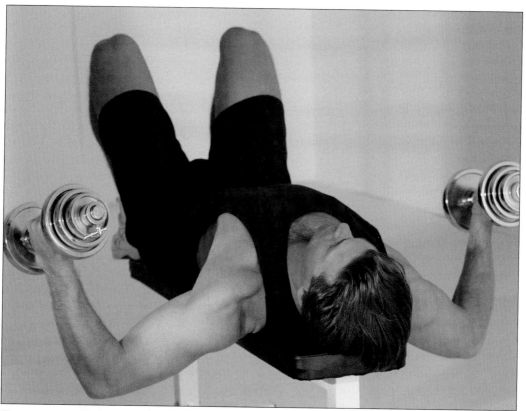

■ **Strength training by doing supersets** *involves performing two or more exercises in a row without stopping to rest between the exercises. Each superset should consist of exercises that work opposing muscle groups, like the chest press (shown) and overhead press.*

Give me a break

SOMETIMES TOO MUCH of a good thing can be, well, not so good. As great as exercise is, it is possible to overtrain. When that happens, your body stops responding in a positive way. How do you know if you're guilty of exercise overindulgence? See if any of these symptoms apply to you:

- You've been exercising frequently, but your regular workout seems more difficult
- Exercise leaves you more exhausted than energized
- Your performance is decreasing despite diligent workouts
- You experience a loss of co-ordination
- It takes you longer to recover from muscle soreness
- You have no appetite
- Your stomach hurts
- You get sick often

In addition, the psychological benefits that come with exercise disappear when you overtrain, so you might feel depressed and apathetic, have difficulty concentrating, or even have reduced self-esteem.

If you've been working out too hard and you feel any of these symptoms, it's time for you to cut back a little or take a break.

Remember – moderation is the key.

If you find yourself exercising beyond the point of exhaustion, while injured, or to the exclusion of other aspects of your life, then it is definitely time to take a break.

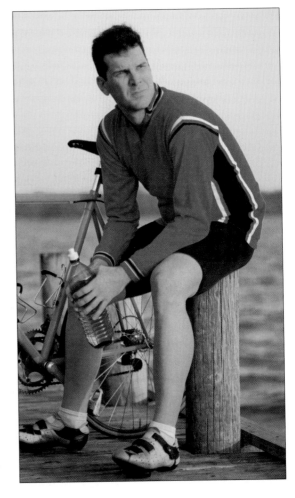

■ **If cycling begins to drain** *rather than revitalize you, consider slowing the pace a little, or even stopping altogether for a short while.*

Lighten the load

If you don't want to stop altogether, then just try lighter workouts for a while. Also, remember that taking a few days off is okay. If you need to take a longer mini-break from exercising, reduce your meal portions so you won't have to worry about putting on weight. Your body doesn't need as much food when you're not exercising.

Muscle won't turn into fat if you stop exercising. Muscle and fat are two separate things. It's like saying your car will turn into a bicycle if you don't drive it.

If you stop for longer than a few weeks, your heart and muscle strength will decrease, but don't let that stop you from jumping right back in when you're ready, albeit at a lesser pace.

A simple summary

✔ After working out for a while, sometimes we hit a plateau. The best thing to do is recognize it and move on.

✔ Take a good look at your progress and goals. Stay flexible and make small changes to your goals if you need to.

✔ The same old workout routine gets boring after a while. Mix in some new moves.

✔ Train like the pros with cross training, interval training, and circuit training, and by using the hard–easy principle and doing supersets.

✔ If you've become obsessed with exercise, maybe it's time to take a break.

✔ If taking a longer break, cut back your food intake to prevent you from gaining weight.

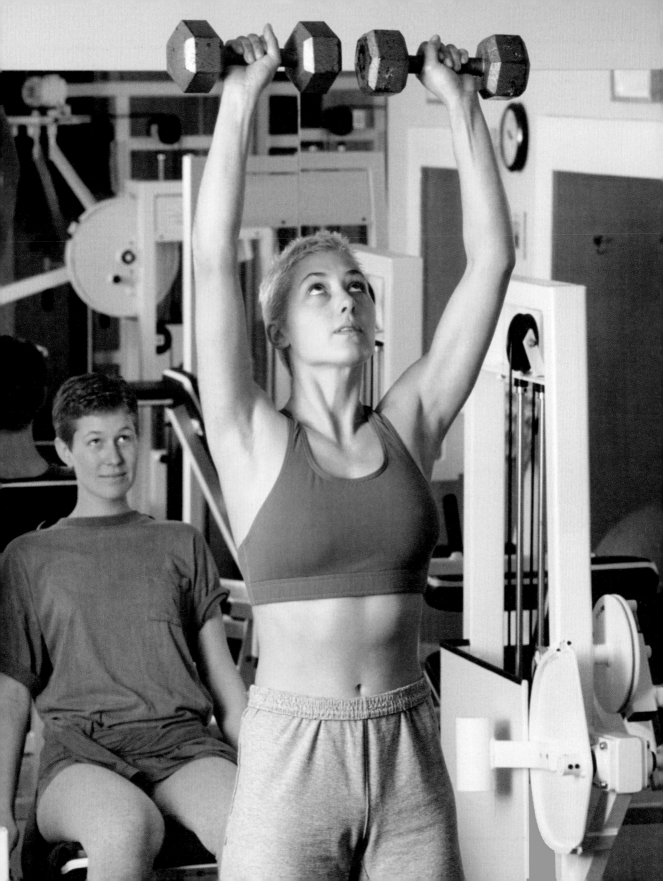

Chapter 19

Let's Assess

A SIMPLE WAY TO MEASURE FITNESS PROGRESS is by comparing your current abilities with your initial assessment. Can you do more push-ups than you could when you first began? Stretch a little further? If so, congratulations! If not, I've included a few tips to help you improve. Lace up your running or walking shoes and get ready to take a new aerobics fitness test to see what your overall level of fitness is now. But be aware of what your body will and won't do. Some factors that affect your body shape, such as genes and gender, are beyond your control. Each individual reacts differently to exercise.

In this chapter...

✔ Progress report

✔ Aerobic fitness challenge

✔ Realistic expectations

YOU'VE BEEN WORKING OUT HARD – WILL YOU PASS YOUR FITNESS TEST?

Progress report

HOW DO YOU KNOW *if you're getting fit? One way to gauge it is by looking at your starting point. Get out your results from the quiz in Chapter 2, and let's do a progress report. If you've added more exercise to your life, then you should be able to measure the results. If it's only been a few weeks, wait until you have at least a month or two under your belt before you retake the test. If you have been exercising but aren't getting the results you want, I've included some simple suggestions to help you improve.*

Is your Body Mass Index within a healthy range?

Step on the scale and recalculate your BMI. (You will recall that you calculated your Body Mass Index in Chapter 2.) Look back in your journal and compare your scores. If your BMI is still too high, try adding at least 30 more minutes of aerobic activity per week. You could fit this in by adding two 15-minute jogs per week, or by signing up for a half-hour-long aerobic fitness class that meets once a week. Or add a few *callisthenics* into your routine. Also, although exercising makes you hungry, make sure that you're not consuming more calories than you're burning. If your BMI is too low, add more strength training to your routine to build muscle. If you haven't already done so, join a gym and take advantage of the free weights and weight machines.

> **DEFINITION**
>
> **Callisthenics** *are exercises that don't require any equipment, such as windmills, jumping jacks, and squat thrusts.*

What is your waist-to-hip ratio?

I hope you didn't throw that measuring tape out of the window after the first test, because I want you to use it again to see how that waist-to-hip ratio is coming along.

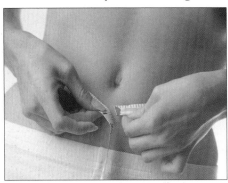

■ **Remeasuring your waist and hips** *will help you assess your progress.*

If your waist-to-hip ratio is in the healthy range, keep it up. If it's still in the borderline or unhealthy range, then you may need to cut more fat and calories out of your diet. Start small; try eating smaller portions for one meal a day. Some people are more likely than others to carry extra weight in the middle. If you're one of those people, then you need to be extra careful because you're more at risk of health problems. Unfair, isn't it? Crunches can certainly help tone up the midsection, but you can't lose weight from one area only. When you lose weight it comes from all over your body.

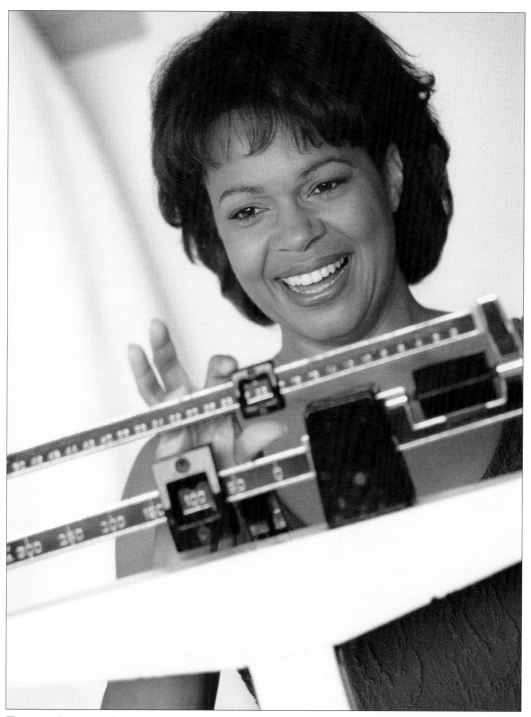

■ **Reweigh yourself** *a month or two into your exercise programme and recalculate your BMI. This will reveal if you're on the right track or if you need to make some adjustments to your workout schedule.*

There's no such thing as "spot-reducing." Getting rid of fat on a specific area of the body just doesn't work.

Are your muscles lean and mean?

It's impossible for one exercise to test all-over muscle strength, but push-ups and crunches are two good indicators. Now that you know how to do the perfect push-up, drop and give me 20! Well, you don't have to do 20, just get down on the floor in push-up position and see how many you can do without stopping. Can you do more than you did when you first started out? If you can, great, you're moving in the right direction. If not, then your upper body needs a little work. Add a few push-ups to your morning routine, or get some light hand weights and lift a few sets while you watch your favourite television show.

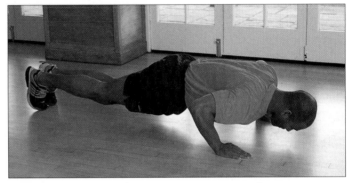

■ **See how many push-ups** *you can manage without stopping. Can you do more than you were able to do before?*

Next, try to do as many crunches as you can without stopping, making sure to maintain good form throughout. Remember not to pull from the neck; and keep the tension in your abs. How did you do? If you can do more than you did for your baseline assessment, well done. If not, the best thing to do is to add a few abdominal exercises to your routine. Go back to Chapter 13 for more on abdominal exercises, and find one you like. If you're not a big fan of crunches and sit-ups, Pilates is another wonderful way to tone the abs.

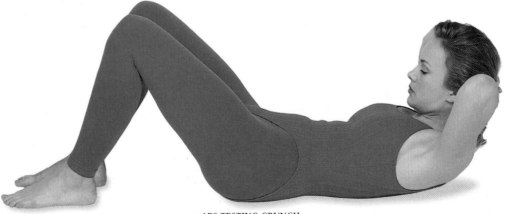

ABS-TESTING CRUNCH

Are you as flexible as a rubber band?

Well, you don't need to be that flexible, but let's see if you've made any progress. Warm up with a brisk walk, jog in place, or dance around the room – you know the routine. Then retake the flexibility test.

Can you reach further than you could before? If not, add more stretching to your day. Try adding a few gentle stretches to your pre-bedtime routine. It feels great and it can help relax you and get you to sleep. Yoga is a great way to increase flexibility. Find out if there's a yoga class in your area or try a yoga video.

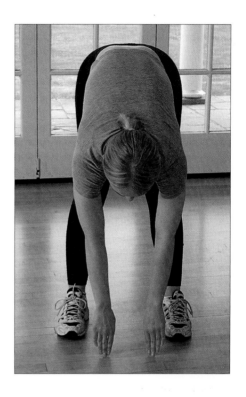

■ **Being able to reach** *and touch the floor is a sign of good flexibility. If your flexibility hasn't improved much, add more stretching to your fitness routine.*

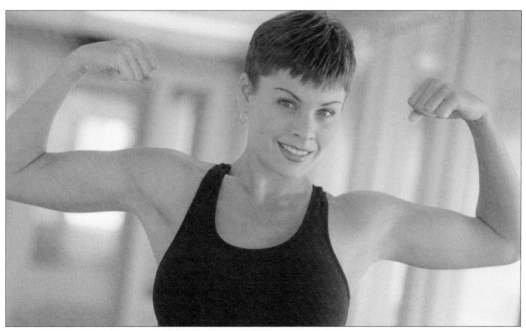

■ **If you're leaner and meaner** *than you were, congratulate yourself! You've made great progress, so make a pledge to keep up the good work – you're well on the way to a new you.*

Aerobic fitness challenge

HERE'S AN OPPORTUNITY TO TEST *your aerobic fitness, which is the best measure of overall fitness. This test can be challenging, so I've saved it for last. It's best to take this test after you've been exercising for a while.*

Take the aerobic fitness test only when you feel ready to run or walk more than a mile.

The purpose of this test, created by the US Cooper Institute for Aerobic Research, is to see how fast you can run, jog, or walk at a steady pace for 3.3 km (1.5 miles) on a flat surface. Your finish time is used to approximate your aerobic fitness. This test is best done outdoors. If you can't run outside for some reason, you can take the aerobic fitness test on a treadmill instead.

Taking the fitness test

Don't eat for 2 hours before this test. Pick a safe flat path or track, and use a stopwatch or a watch with a second hand to see how long it takes you to cover 3.3 km (1.5 miles), which is six laps around a typical half-kilometre (quarter-mile) running track. If you don't think you can run the entire distance, start out walking and then try to build up to running later in the course. Pace yourself and use caution in how hard you push yourself. Although you want to do your best, you should feel only tired at the end, rather than nauseous or weak.

Before you begin, warm up for a few minutes by walking around; you should also walk for a few minutes after finishing the test.

■ **Make sure you warm up** *properly before the test by walking briskly for a few minutes.*

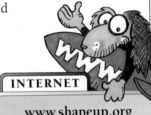

INTERNET

www.shapeup.org

This is the official web site for Shape Up America! It offers information on exercise and nutrition, plus various fitness assessment tests at /fitness/assess/fset2.htm. These results are based on your age, height, and weight. Find the one that is the closest match to you. If you want an exact calculation, go to this web site after you've timed your run or walk, and put in your age, height, weight, and gender.

HOW DO YOU MEASURE UP?

Compare your time for the 3.3 km (1.5-mile) walk or run with the results below by finding the closest match to you. For an exact calculation, go to www.shapeup.org.

WOMEN

Age	Time	Fitness level
25	Below 12:51 12:51 to 14:35 14:36 to 16:26 16:27 and above	Superior Moderate Minimal Unfit
35	Below 13:44 13:44 to 15:20 15:21 to 16:58 16:59 and above	Superior Moderate Minimal Unfit
45	Below 14:33 14:33 to 16:12 16:13 to 17:29 17:30 and above	Superior Moderate Minimal Unfit

MEN

Age	Time	Fitness level
25	Below 10:16 10:16 to 11:49 11:50 to 13:53 13:54 and above	Superior Moderate Minimal Unfit
35	Below 10:48 10:48 to 12:38 12:39 to 14:24 14:25 and above	Superior Moderate Minimal Unfit
45	Below 11:45 11:45 to 13:22 13:23 to 15:26 15:27 and above	Superior Moderate Minimal Unfit

VO2 max

The VO2 max is another measure of aerobic fitness. The definition of VO2 max is the maximal rate at which oxygen can be consumed per minute. This is an excellent measure of overall fitness. It's frequently used by endurance athletes, but it's a good indicator for everyone.

VO2 max is the maximum ability of the body to transport oxygen from the air to the muscles for energy generation. It involves the heart's capacity to pump oxygen-rich blood to the muscles, as well as the muscles' efficiency in extracting and utilizing the oxygen. VO2 max is measured in milliliters of oxygen per kilogram of body weight per minute of exercise (ml/kg/min).

If the arteries and veins are like roads, and doing aerobic exercise is like paving those roads (as mentioned in Chapter 1), so the oxygenated blood can get around easier, then having a high VO2 max means your veins and arteries are like a motorway. VO2 max is a measure of how quickly that oxygenated blood can get to the muscles.

Testing VO2

In general, the higher your VO2 max, the better your overall fitness. Although genetic factors establish the boundaries of your VO2 max, exercise can improve it, and endurance training in particular can push the limits of those boundaries. Elite athletes have the highest VO2 max. The range of VO2 max is 20 to 90. An elite endurance athlete might have a VO2 max around 70 and a sedentary person's would be somewhere around 35. It's fairly expensive to get your VO2 max tested, and you don't really need to unless you are a serious endurance athlete who needs precise numbers.

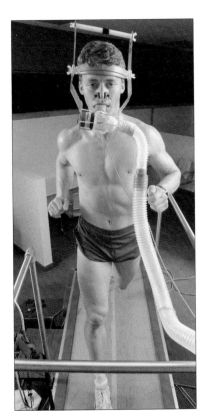

THE VO2 MAX TEST

> **Trivia...**
>
> *The record for the highest VO2 max goes to a Norwegian cross-country skier who had a VO2 max of 94 ml/kg/min.*

The test involves a long, exhaustive run on a treadmill while connected to a respiration unit and heart-rate monitor. There are also easier tests, such as a written quiz that asks you what your daily physical activity level is and estimates your VO2 max from that. There is a written quiz like this also on www.shapeup.org.

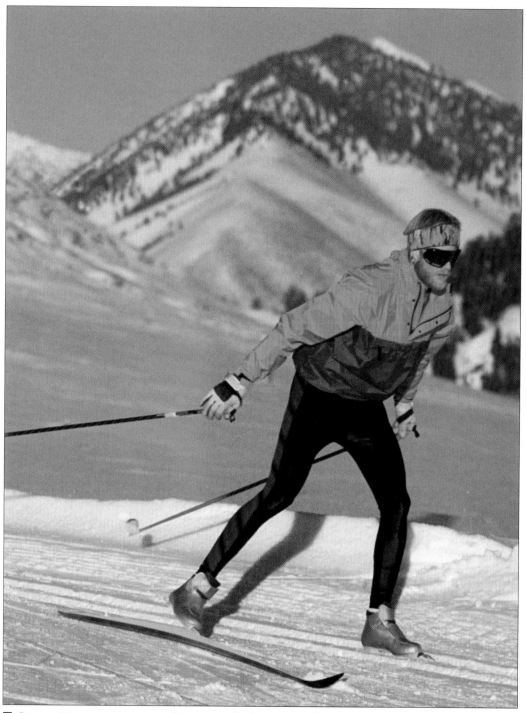

■ **Competitive cross-country skiers** *generally have very high measures of VO2 max. This means that they are extremely fit; their bodies are able to process and circulate oxygen with optimum efficiency.*

Realistic expectations

AS YOU MOVE ALONG THE PATH to fitness, it's important to remember that your personal physique will respond to exercise in its own unique way. In truth, there is only so much you can do to change what you're born with; your body type, your VO2 max to some extent, and, of course, gender are some things that are impossible to change through exercises. Keep in mind the limitations imposed by nature as you begin exercising as well as once you've been exercising regularly.

Some things you can't change

Fitness is an individual quality that varies from person to person. It's influenced by age, sex, heredity, personal habits, and eating practices. Exercise can make anyone more fit, but it will affect everyone a bit differently. Every body will respond in a unique way. Don't compare yourself with anyone else, even if it's your workout partner and you're doing all the same workouts. There are some things we can't change. There's the VO2 max, for example – we can raise it to some extent, but everyone has a different threshold. Some people naturally have higher VO2 maxes than others.

Also, you may have noticed that some people seem to be able to eat whatever they want and not gain any weight, while others eat salads but can't get rid of a stomach paunch. Some people have naturally higher metabolisms than others. Be aware of that and don't get discouraged.

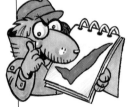

It can be frustrating when someone who hasn't been working out at all can lift more weight than I can, but it just makes me want to try harder.

Gender role in fitness

There have been many discussions and arguments about the differences between men's and women's capacities for fitness. Fortunately, many old myths claiming that it is unhealthy for women to exercise have been dispelled. Women were banned from running marathons for many years, for example, because people thought that long-distance running could displace the uterus, or cause women to develop large manly muscles.

Trivia...

Kathrine Switzer set the pace for women runners worldwide in the Boston Marathon in 1967. Women were banned from running marathons at the time and a race official tried to stop her, saying, "You don't belong here!" But she did belong: she went on to run 35 marathons, and won the 1974 New York City Marathon.

Physical differences

While we all know by now that women can and often do excel in athletics, there are real differences between men's and women's bodies. As I've mentioned, women's muscles don't bulk up as much as men's. This is a good thing, because most men want to bulk up, and most women want to be toned and svelte. Although there are exceptions, other differences are that most women are smaller than most men, and women have a greater amount of body fat. On the flip side, women are often more flexible.

The bottom line is: focus on the things you can change – eating habits, exercise, and personal habits – and don't worry about things you can't change. Exercise and realize your unique body's potential for fitness.

■ **Long-distance running** *is no longer dominated by men; many women excel in this field. However, if a man and a woman pursued the same training schedule, their bodies would be affected differently.*

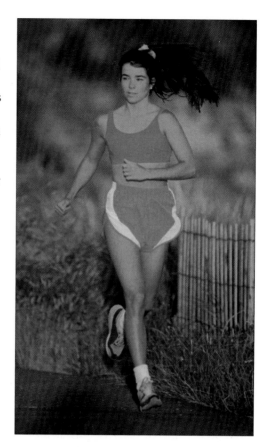

A simple summary

✔ A retake of the fitness quiz from the beginning of the book will show you how you're coming along in your fitness programme.

✔ It's important to realize that every body is different, so don't be tempted to compare yourself with anyone else.

✔ Aerobic fitness is one of the best measures of overall fitness. Take the aerobic assessment tests here, and find out how fit you are.

✔ Learn to accept that there are plenty of things you can change, but some that you can't.

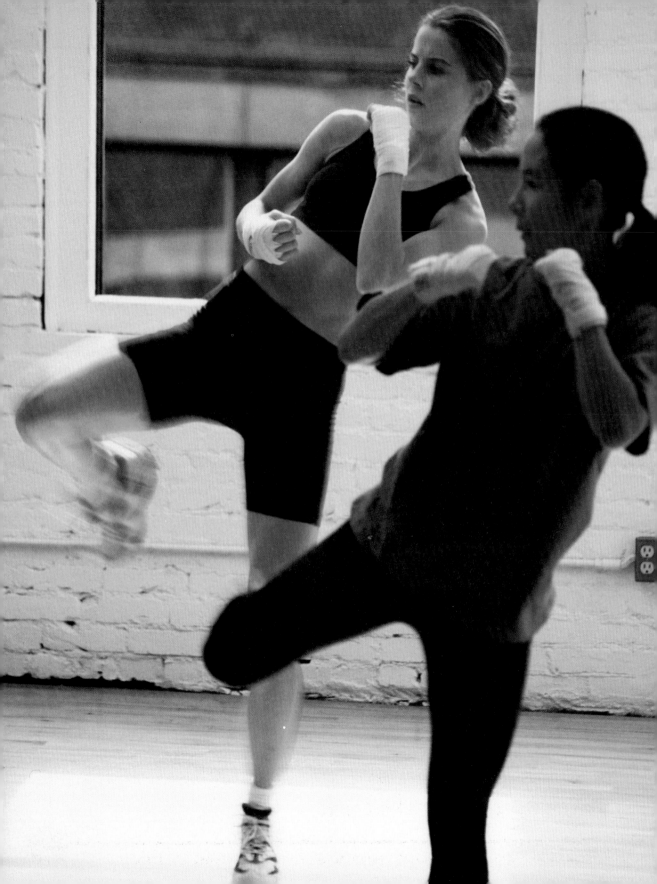

Chapter 20

What's Next?

WHAT ARE THE NEXT TRENDS IN FITNESS? We'll see more focus on the mind-body-spirit connection, balance work, and core training, to name a few. As young and old continue to look to alternative ways to get healthy, influences from India and China continue to infiltrate the world of fitness in the West. Most important is that you find exercise you like.

In this chapter...

✓ Future fitness trends

✓ More Eastern influence

✓ Balance and core training

✓ Funky options

✓ Keeping your fitness habit, whatever the trend

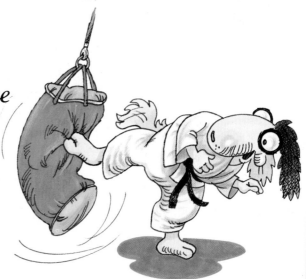

EXPERIMENT WITH DIFFERENT TYPES OF EXERCISE AND YOU'RE BOUND TO FIND SOMETHING YOU LIKE

Future fitness trends

THE BIGGEST TREND IN FITNESS *these days is devising exercises or disciplines that forge the mind-body-spirit connection. Many people are realizing the importance of balancing a healthy body with a healthy mind and spirit.*

Fitness in general seems to be moving away from straight-up exercise and into creating a well-rounded person, not just well-rounded biceps. Even within the physical realm, there is an increasing emphasis on balance and inner (literally inner, as in the deepest muscle layers) strength. I know plenty of ex-aerobic junkies who have turned to more contemplative exercise like yoga or Pilates, and who swear that they feel better all-round.

One woman who taught aerobics for years and now owns a yoga studio says she couldn't even sit through an entire movie when she was doing aerobics, but now she can meditate for hours. She attributes her new calmness to yoga.

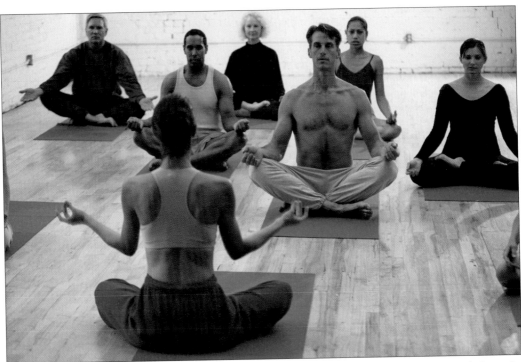

■ **Yoga has attracted many devotees** *thanks to its reputation for promoting both mental and physical wellbeing. Many yoga postures emphasize deep breathing, relaxed movement, and concentration.*

More Eastern influence

EASTERN DISCIPLINES *such as yoga and tai chi are becoming increasingly popular. They've been around for years in India and China, but the West is still just catching on. Qigong and other martial arts have also been around for many years, and there's currently a surge of renewed interest in these.*

Qigong

Qigong (*chi kung*) is an ancient Chinese healing art that combines movement and meditation with deep breathing. It has been used for 2,000 years in China as a way to cure disease and promote health. It's being used more frequently in countries outside of China as exercise and therapy.

> **DEFINITION**
>
> *Qi (like chi) means energy and gong means skill.* **Qigong** *is the skill of attracting vital energy.*

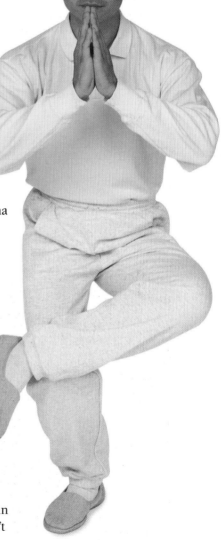

A QIGONG POSE

There are many different kinds of qigong. It seems a little strange to call something that has been around for 2,000 years a "future trend", but the popularity of qigong is growing exponentially. Evidence of this growing popularity is the World Tai Chi and Qigong Day. Born in 1997, World Tai Chi and Qigong Day takes place in public parks in 80 countries. On this day in April, large groups gather in public parks at 10am local time to perform tai chi and qigong. Observation of this day starts on the east coast of Australia and ends in Hawaii. The exact figure isn't known, but about 50,000 people participate.

> **INTERNET**
>
> **www.worldtaichiday.org**
>
> *This is the web site for World Tai Chi and Qigong Day. To find out more about it and how to get involved, log on here.*

313

Popular martial arts

Here are some simple definitions of commonly found martial arts:

a **Karate:** this is a Japanese art of self-defence and fighting without weapons. You strike with your hands, elbows, knees, and feet. You use punching, striking, and blocking techniques, making the most of the laws of physics to increase the damage by each blow. Karate emphasizes a solid stance and footing, so punching and striking are used more often than kicking. Karate means "empty hands", which refers to using no weapons and having a clear mind

b **Tae kwon do:** this is a Korean art of self-defence. It's similar to karate, but there's a stronger emphasis on foot technique. This martial art specializes in fast, high, and spinning kicks. Bare hands and feet are used instead of weapons. Modern tae kwon do is influenced by Japanese karate because Japan dominated Korea from 1910 until the end of World War II. Tae kwon do has a military background, and a code of honour that includes such sentiments as "be faithful to your spouse" and "never retreat in battle", among others

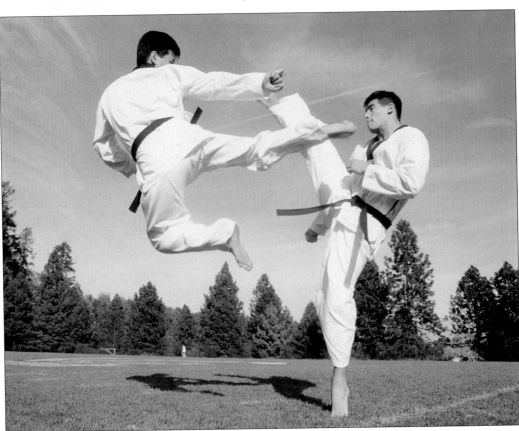

TAE KWON DO HIGH KICKS

c **Kung fu:** this Chinese martial art is similar to karate. It's one of the earliest and longest surviving sports. Kung fu entails various forms of fighting that include using fists, weapons, kicking, hitting, throwing, holding, chopping, and thrusting. Sound like fun? Better hope your opponent is small

d **Judo:** judo is a Japanese sport and method of training similar to wrestling. It was developed in the late 19th century using the principles of balance and leverage adapted from jujitsu. It's also known as the "gentle way", and is a popular Olympic sport

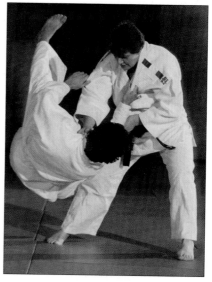

JUDO WRESTLING

e **Aikido:** this is a Japanese self-defence system that resembles the fighting methods of jujitsu and judo in its utilization of twisting and throwing techniques. Aikido was developed in the 1930s and 1940s as a technique that incorporates self-defence, spiritual enlightenment, physical health, and peace of mind. It focuses on using your opponent's own energy to gain control over them and then throwing them away from you rather than punching and kicking as in karate and tae kwon do. This martial art aims for harmony and is co-operative, not competitive

f **Hapkido:** the goal of this Korean martial art is not to meet your opponent's force with direct force, but to redirect it using a circular motion and then counter-attacking with a powerful combination of circular techniques. It uses joint locking, throws, take-downs, and dynamic kicking techniques, strikes, and punches similar to those of tae kwon do. Even at the beginning level, meditation is used. It's mentally and physically challenging. The Korean names for the techniques are used to keep a sense of tradition

g **Capoeira:** this is a martial art discipline that comes not from Asia but from Africa via Brazil. Capoeira was created by African slaves in Brazil about 400 years ago. It's a combination of dancing, fighting, gymnastics, and music. The slaves had to disguise what they were doing, which is how dance came into it. It involves an impressive combination of cartwheels, kicks, and somersaults. The unique style brings together beauty and power, and develops mental and physical balance, physical conditioning, self-defence, music, and art. It's a stylized dance practised in a circle, with the music usually provided by people inside the circle playing instruments. It uses kicks and leg sweeps for attacks and evasive dodges for defence

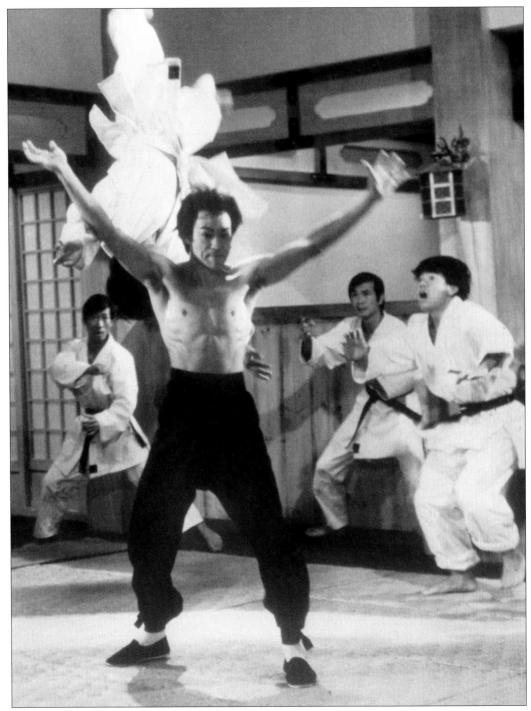

■ **Bruce Lee** *starred in more than 30 action films and became known as the 20th century's greatest martial artist. He developed his own flexible yet practical martial arts style, called jeet kune do.*

Jujitsu: also spelled jiujitsu or jujutsu, this ancient martial art has been around since about 255 BC. Modern jujitsu is a fighting and self-defence art for anyone regardless of physical conditioning. Jujitsu is suitable for men and women of all shapes and sizes. It places priority on practising self-defence without competition rules or regulations. Kicks, punches, elbows, throws – you basically do anything to protect yourself. It's an excellent form of exercise that increases strength, endurance, and flexibility

> ### Trivia...
> Popular action star of yesteryear, Bruce Lee, studied jujitsu before he developed his own style.

Other martial arts

Martial arts have always had fans outside the Asian countries from which they originated. There are hundreds of different kinds of martial arts. Most martial arts, such as karate, judo, or tae kwon do, take a certain amount of strength, a lot of discipline, and time. A martial art is more than just exercise; it often involves honour, respect, and tradition.

Although practising any form of martial arts is a great way to get strong and flexible, it's best to be in decent shape before embarking upon a physically and mentally challenging martial art. You'll find some elements of the martial arts can be found in fitness classes offered at your local gym. Kickboxing aerobics is a very popular workout that incorporates physical elements of martial arts in a fitness class that anyone can enjoy (without having to battle an opponent!).

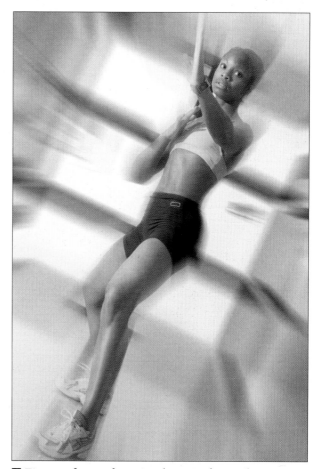

■ **Fitness classes** *featuring elements of martial arts are becoming increasing popular, particularly with women.*

Martial arts are an excellent way to make that mind-body-spirit connection that so many people desire.

Striking and grappling

Although there are numerous variations of martial arts, they can basically be broken down into two groups: the striking arts, such as karate, tae kwon do, and kung fu, which involve punching and kicking, and the grappling arts, such as judo and aikido, which incorporate holds and throwing. You need a partner for the grappling arts. Jujitsu and hapkido combine the two groups, as they use both striking and grappling.

Before you sign up for a martial arts class, evaluate your fitness goals. Martial arts builds strength and stamina for quick powerful bursts of activity instead of the endurance that marathoners have or the muscles of a body builder.

Once you get started on your fitness programme and feel quite good, look into the different kinds of martial arts classes and see which one best suits you. Observe a few classes to gauge the level of contact involved and the level of fitness required, and to find a teacher you'd like to work with.

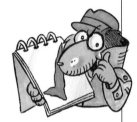

Yoga and ayurveda

It's no secret that growing numbers of people are incorporating yoga into their fitness routines. It's not just for people who live in communes any more! Yoga classes are now being held at leisure centres and gyms everywhere. While some yoga classes are true to the original Indian forms (there are many different kinds), many are getting a Western makeover. A popular class that could soon be on the way here from the US is disco yoga – you probably wouldn't find that in an *ashram* in India.

> **DEFINITION**
>
> **Ashram** *is the traditional Indian name for yoga center.*

Along with yoga, another Indian import that has been gaining popularity in the West is ayurveda, a 5,000-year-old health-care science. I see it referred to regarding everything from yoga moves to health or beauty products. Ayurveda combines the physical, spiritual, and emotional being. Ayurveda views life as an interrelationship between physical processes and external factors and emotions. Health is maintained by the balance of three energies present in all living things.

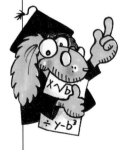

According to ayurvedic principles, the three energies, or doshas, that must be balanced for health are: kapha, which is earth and matter; vata, which is air and movement; and pitta, which is fire and transformation.

IDENTIFYING YOUR PRIMARY DOSHA

Some people take the notion of doshas a step further and say that everyone has a primary dosha that is determined by their energy level and their emotional being. Being aware of your primary dosha can help you balance your exercise and even your life. Identify whether you're a vata, pitta, or kapha type to see which types of exercise might most benefit you.

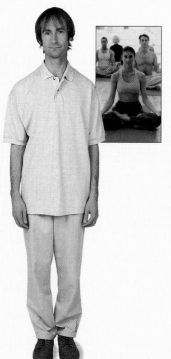

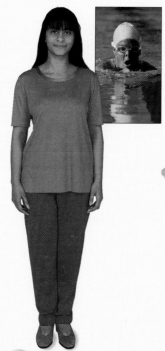

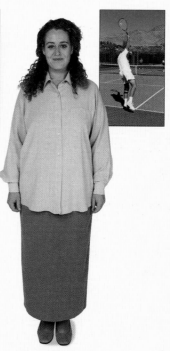

1 Vata

Vata types may be tall or short and of slight build; they are creative with quick, nervous movements, but they tend to waste energy in quick bursts. These types would benefit from adding some calming workouts, such as yoga or tai chi, into their routines.

2 Pitta

Pitta types are of average height and even proportions; confident and ambitious, they can be aggressively competitive. They tend to be like middle-distance runners with good reserves, and could benefit from fun, mellow workouts like swimming or cycling.

3 Kapha

Kapha types are heavily built, slow-moving, and physically strong; they are stable and patient, but they are inclined towards possessiveness. They tend towards wanting to sit on the couch and could enrich their exercise lives with some aerobics, running, or tennis.

Balance and core training

THESE DAYS, BALANCE WORK *is quickly taking its place alongside endurance, flexibility, and strength training as another important building block for a complete fitness programme. Balance work is what it sounds like – practising keeping your balance. Core training has also hit the fitness scene in a big way as a way of strengthening the body's deepest muscles.*

Balance work can include activities like walking on an imaginary tightrope on the ground, or balancing on one leg with your eyes open or shut. Many sports teams are incorporating this kind of exercise into their practices.

Imagine a basketball player with a poor sense of balance trying to recover after catching an elbow or after reaching at an impossible angle to get a rebound. Balance training forces you to use muscles that stabilize your body, especially those in your core.

Professional basketball players, The New York Knicks, use balance training in practice to give them an edge.

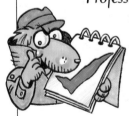

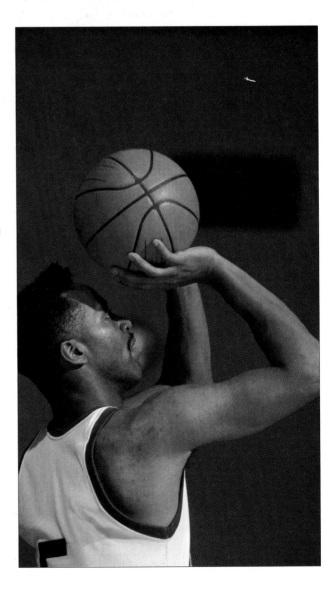

■ **Balance work** *is now an important aspect of training for many professional athletes, including basketball players.*

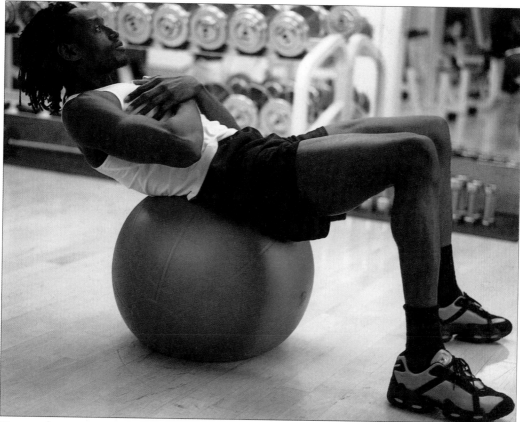

■ **Core training** *involves strengthening the deepest muscle layers, rather than just the superficial muscles. It can help you improve your power, balance, and strength.*

Working your core

As spinning and step become rather old hat, albeit remaining as gym class mainstays, the new trend of "core training" is coming up to take their place in the spotlight. More and more classes, exercise videos, and training techniques mention working your core. I see this word popping up everywhere in the fitness world. *Core* training pops up in yoga classes, sports, and strength training.

> **DEFINITION**
>
> *Your **core** comprises the muscles that stabilize your torso, including the muscles of the abs and the lower back.*

Most training and conditioning focuses on the superficial muscles that move our arms and legs, but strong core muscles – the deepest muscle layers – are central to movement. Focusing on them can improve all-round strength. Strengthening your core, and thereby improving your power, balance, and strength, is good for everyone from the professional athlete to the average person.

Funky options

THERE ARE ALWAYS *new and different ways to get fit popping up in trendy health clubs and gyms. People are forever looking for exciting and non-traditional ways to get in shape and have fun.*

Some interesting classes I've come across lately are the aforementioned disco yoga – yoga with a disco ball hanging from the ceiling and a turntable playing old disco records. There's also circus training in which you do handstands, backbends, and somersaults, learn to juggle, hang from a trapeze, and form a human pyramid.

Trivia...

Even the corporate world has been swept up by the fun of the circus. Companies are now organizing training workshops so that staff can brush up on their circus skills. Apparently, learning juggling, static and flying trapeze, acrobatics, and clowning helps promote self-development, build confidence, inspire team spirit, and improve co-ordination and fitness.

There are exercises with a new twist, like basketball aerobics and underwater kickboxing. Also, many people are now getting into "rebounding", which is jumping on a small trampoline, a surface that is particularly forgiving on the joints. In other words, if you can think of it, it's probably out there.

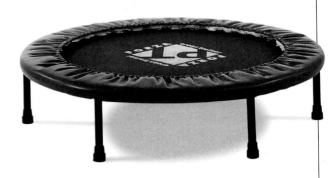

■ **Jumping on a small trampoline** *or "rebounding" is good aerobic exercise and very gentle on the joints. It's great for balance and co-ordination, but best of all, it's fun.*

Keeping your fitness habit, whatever the trend

ANOTHER TREND *in the health and fitness arena is that women are no longer the only ones who have strong societal pressure to look good. Men these days are "supposed" to be every bit as concerned with their appearance as women. As for women, the trend is toward more aggressive exercise. But trends come and go. The most important thing is that you find something that you enjoy, that you will stick to.*

The gender trends

The popularity of the movie, *The Full Monty*, shows how men can be seen as "objects" too, and can stress and worry about a couple of extra inches around the waist. Also, while popular dolls for girls have long been portraying women with impossible proportions, lately male dolls have developed giant muscles. This trend has led to more men taking steroids and other supplements to build up to these expectations. This is a very dangerous habit.

Steer clear of steroids or any other supplements to bulk you up. Many of these can be unhealthy and even dangerous.

Not only are more women enrolling in the popular kickboxing classes, they are also taking up boxing. Also, opportunities for women to play professional competitive sports continue to grow.

Television reflects this trend also, with heroines like Xena the Warrior Princess and Buffy the Vampire Slayer – beautiful women who can beat up the bad guy with style. The trend is for women not only to look good, but to be able to high-kick the enemy in a blink of an eye.

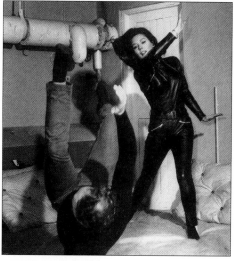

■ **The Avengers'** *hard-hitting, leather-clad Emma Peel (played by Diana Rigg) was one of the first all-action heroines symbolizing glamorous toughness.*

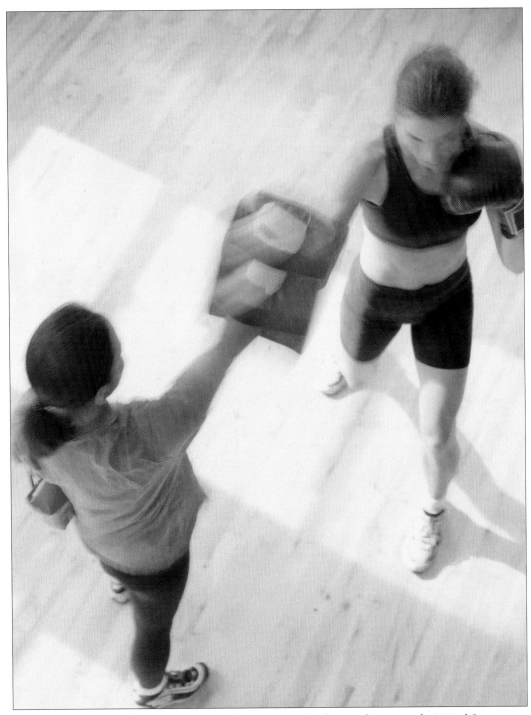

■ **Boxing classes for women** *are all set to become as popular here as they are in the United States, where vast numbers of lady boxers have found that this strenuous workout is a great way to get rid of stress.*

Of course, the television heroines aren't realistic role models, but this kind of strong-woman attitude has seeped into the fitness world as reflected in the popularity of kickboxing, boxing, and other classes that promote strength and power.

Commit to staying fit

If everyone around you is touting the glories of yoga, for example, but you really don't enjoy it, find something else. There is something out there for everyone. The good thing about trends is that you might be exposed to something new you hadn't thought of. Try a new class, try a new sport; you might discover a hidden talent! Experiment and try new things; do whatever it takes to keep yourself interested and involved. Don't let fitness be a fleeting trend for you, make it a part of your lifestyle.

Keep looking for new ways to stay fit. Listen to your body, keep it simple, and remember – have fun!

A simple summary

✔ Balance work, and connecting the mind, body, and spirit are now popular elements of fitness programmes.

✔ Many people find martial arts, such as tai chi, qigong, karate, or tae kwon do, great ways to get physically and mentally fit.

✔ Training the core muscles and enhancing balancing skills are slowly becoming standard fitness fodder.

✔ Power yoga? Circus training? Rebounding? There are all kinds of fun classes and training regimens to keep exercise exciting.

✔ Fitness trends reflect the changing roles of gender and body image.

✔ Just because fitness trends come and go, don't let fitness go! Staying fit is a lifelong commitment.

Fitness log

DATE	_/_/_	_/_/_	_/_/_	_/_/_
My weight				
My height				
My BMI (body mass index)				
My waist-to-hip ratio				

MY MEASUREMENTS

Chest				
Arms				
Thigh				
Waist				
Hips				
Calf				

MUSCLE STRENGTH

No. of push-ups				
No. of crunches				

FLEXIBILITY

Floor test (note how far you can reach)				
Shoulder test (note how far you can reach)				

DATE	_/_/_	_/_/_	_/_/_	_/_/_
AEROBIC FITNESS				
My maximum heart rate				
My target heart rate				
Time for 1.5 mile (3.2 km) run				

MY FITNESS GOALS

Long-term goals

	Milestones	Date	Goal	Reward
1				
2				
3				
4				
5				

NOTES

Exercise diary

WEEK __ : MONDAY   DATE __/__/__

Warm-up [ ]   Stretches [ ]   Duration

WEIGHTS

Exercise	Set 1		Set 2		Set 3		Set 4		Set 5	
	Planned	Actual	Planned	Actual	Planned	Actual	Planned	Actual	Planned	Actual

Remember to include no. of reps and weight for example, 8/40kg   Duration

NOTES

Warm-up	☐	Stretches	☐	Duration

CARDIOVASCULAR

Exercise	Duration	
	Planned	Actual

NUTRITION

Breakfast	
Mid-morning	
Lunch	
Mid-afternoon	
Dinner	
Late evening	
Snacks	

NOTES

Exercise diary

WEEK ___ : TUESDAY   DATE __/__/__

| Warm-up | ☐ | Stretches | ☐ | Duration |

WEIGHTS

Exercise	Set 1		Set 2		Set 3		Set 4		Set 5	
	Planned	Actual	Planned	Actual	Planned	Actual	Planned	Actual	Planned	Actual

Remember to include no. of reps and weight for example, 8/40kg   Duration

NOTES

| Warm-up | ☐ | Stretches | ☐ | Duration |

CARDIOVASCULAR

Exercise	Duration	
	Planned	Actual

NUTRITION

Breakfast	
Mid-morning	
Lunch	
Mid-afternoon	
Dinner	
Late evening	
Snacks	

NOTES

Exercise diary

WEEK __ : WEDNESDAY   DATE __/__/__

Warm-up ☐   Stretches ☐   Duration

WEIGHTS

Exercise	Set 1		Set 2		Set 3		Set 4		Set 5	
	Planned	Actual	Planned	Actual	Planned	Actual	Planned	Actual	Planned	Actual

Remember to include no. of reps and weight for example, 8/40kg   Duration

NOTES

Warm-up	☐	Stretches	☐	Duration

CARDIOVASCULAR

Exercise	Duration	
	Planned	Actual

NUTRITION

Breakfast	
Mid-morning	
Lunch	
Mid-afternoon	
Dinner	
Late evening	
Snacks	

NOTES

Exercise diary

WEEK __ : THURSDAY   DATE __/__/__

Warm-up	☐	Stretches	☐	Duration

WEIGHTS

Exercise	Set 1		Set 2		Set 3		Set 4		Set 5	
	Planned	Actual	Planned	Actual	Planned	Actual	Planned	Actual	Planned	Actual

Remember to include no. of reps and weight for example, 8/40kg | Duration

NOTES

Warm-up	☐	Stretches	☐	Duration

CARDIOVASCULAR

Exercise	Duration	
	Planned	Actual

NUTRITION

Breakfast	
Mid-morning	
Lunch	
Mid-afternoon	
Dinner	
Late evening	
Snacks	

NOTES

Exercise diary

WEEK ___ : FRIDAY   DATE ___/___/___

Warm-up ☐   Stretches ☐   Duration

WEIGHTS

Exercise	Set 1		Set 2		Set 3		Set 4		Set 5	
	Planned	Actual	Planned	Actual	Planned	Actual	Planned	Actual	Planned	Actual

Remember to include no. of reps and weight for example, 8/40kg   Duration

NOTES

Warm-up	☐	Stretches	☐	Duration

CARDIOVASCULAR

Exercise	Duration	
	Planned	Actual

NUTRITION

Breakfast	
Mid-morning	
Lunch	
Mid-afternoon	
Dinner	
Late evening	
Snacks	

NOTES

Exercise diary

WEEK __ : SATURDAY   DATE __/__/__

Warm-up	☐	Stretches	☐	Duration

WEIGHTS

Exercise	Set 1		Set 2		Set 3		Set 4		Set 5	
	Planned	Actual	Planned	Actual	Planned	Actual	Planned	Actual	Planned	Actual

Remember to include no. of reps and weight for example, 8/40kg	Duration

NOTES

Warm-up	☐	Stretches	☐	Duration

CARDIOVASCULAR

Exercise	Duration	
	Planned	Actual

NUTRITION

Breakfast	
Mid-morning	
Lunch	
Mid-afternoon	
Dinner	
Late evening	
Snacks	

NOTES

Exercise diary

WEEK __ : SUNDAY   DATE __/__/__

Warm-up	☐	Stretches	☐	Duration

WEIGHTS

Exercise	Set 1		Set 2		Set 3		Set 4		Set 5	
	Planned	Actual	Planned	Actual	Planned	Actual	Planned	Actual	Planned	Actual

Remember to include no. of reps and weight for example, 8/40kg   Duration

NOTES

Warm-up	☐	Stretches	☐	Duration

CARDIOVASCULAR

Exercise	Duration	
	Planned	Actual

NUTRITION

Breakfast	
Mid-morning	
Lunch	
Mid-afternoon	
Dinner	
Late evening	
Snacks	

NOTES

Glossary

Abdominal muscles The large group of muscles running along the front and side of the trunk. Also called "abs".

Aerobic exercise Activity that is sustained, repetitive, or rhythmic, that uses big muscle groups, and that is fairly light to heavy in intensity. Aerobic exercise strengthens the heart.

Aerobics Choreographed fitness classes done to music. Aerobic exercises raise the heart rate.

Alexander Technique A method that works to strip away harmful movement habits and to reduce tension and stress.

Anaerobic Means "without oxygen". It refers to how your muscles work when you exercise so hard that no more oxygen can get to them. Without oxygen muscles burn glycogen for energy.

Arteries Blood vessels that carry blood away from the heart. They're small and strong and bear the highest blood pressure.

Asanas The physical postures of yoga.

Body Mass Index BMI measures your height and weight to determine your body fat.

Callisthenics Exercises that don't require any equipment; these include windmills, jumping jacks, and squat thrusts.

Calorie A unit of energy-producing potential equal to the amount of heat that is contained in food, and released when combined with oxygen from the body. In other words, burning calories means converting food into energy. When you burn calories, the food is used up and isn't stored as fat in the body.

Cardiac muscles Involuntary muscles that govern heart action and also work around the heart.

Cardiovascular "Cardio" means heart, and "vascular" means vessel, or a hollow receptacle for liquid – in this case vascular refers to the vessels that blood moves through. Cardiovascular exercise is exercise that gets your heart beating faster. This in turn gets your blood flowing, circulating more fresh (oxygenated) blood through your body.

Chi In Chinese philosophy, chi is the life force or vital energy.

Concentric contraction A contraction that occurs when two ends of a muscle are brought together.

Core The muscles that stabilize the torso.

Crunch An exercise in which you lift your head, shoulders, and upper back while your lower back stays on the floor.

Dumbbells Hand weights, or free weights, designed to be held in one hand.

Double Dutch A skipping game in which two people crisscross two ropes.

Eccentric contraction A contraction in which two ends of a muscle move apart.

Endorphin A substance used by the nervous system. Endorphins are composed of amino acids. They are made by the pituitary gland and go to the nervous system to reduce pain. They produce effects like those of morphine.

Fartlek training Fartlek is a Swedish word that means "speed play". Fartlek training is a kind of interval training.

Fast-twitch muscles Muscle fibres that contract quickly and that are involved in quick movements.

Feldenkrais Method A method of bringing awareness to the body via gentle movement and directed attention.

Fly A weightlifting term that refers to any lift in which the arms move away from the body.

Gluteus maximus The large muscle that runs along the backside.

Hamstring   The group of muscles and tendons running behind the knee and thigh.

Isometric contraction   A type of muscle contraction in which the length of the muscle doesn't alter but is placed against a resistance, as in arm wrestling.

Lacto-vegetarians   Vegetarians who eat dairy but no eggs or meat, fish, poultry, or seafood.

Meridians   In Chinese philosophy, channels in the body through which the chi, or life force, flows.

Moisture wicking   Refers to the feature in fabrics that helps remove excess moisture from the body.

Out and back run   A training technique that runners use to improve endurance for the second half of a race. You run out for a set amount of time, then turn around and run back, trying to get back faster than it took to go out. Besides improving late-stage endurance, an "out and back" run teaches you to pace yourself during a race.

Overload   An overload is a harder, more-intense-than-average workout.

Ovo-lacto vegetarians   Vegetarians who eat dairy and eggs but no meat, fish, poultry, or seafood.

Plié   A ballet move in which the knees are bent while the back is held straight.

Plyometric training   Exercise to enhance explosive power. It involves a lot of jumping.

Powerhouse   In Pilates, the area just below your belt line.

Pronation   To "pronate" is to turn or rotate the sole of the foot so that the inner edge of the sole bears the body's weight. Pronation refers to the way your foot rotates when you run.

Qigong   A Chinese healing art that loosely translates as "attracting energy".

Quadriceps   Also called "quads", these are the muscles in the front of the thigh.

Recumbent   Recumbent means reclining. On a recumbent bike or a recumbent stair climber, the exercise is done in a seated position, with legs out in front (instead of below).

Rep   Rep is short for repetition; it refers to one full range of motion.

Resistance band   A long rubber tube or band used for resistance exercise.

Set   A cluster of repetitions.

Skeletal muscles   The voluntary movement muscles that we tone and shape when we exercise.

Slow-twitch muscles   Slow-twitch muscle fibres contract more slowly than fast-twitch ones, are heartier (don't fatigue as easily), and are used mostly in endurance exercises.

Smooth muscles   These line the walls of internal organs (excluding the heart) and work involuntarily.

Spa cuisine   Healthful food that is low in fat and calories.

Stability ball   A large rubber ball used to develop strength, flexibility, and balance. Also called a fitness ball or a Swiss ball.

Strength training   Exercise that involves weight-bearing or resistance exercise.

Talk test   An easy way for a beginner to assess if he or she is working out too hard. If you can't easily carry on a conversation while exercising, slow down.

Tantien   The area just below the navel. It's considered the centre of the body's life force. (See "chi".)

Target heart rate   What your heart rate should be while you're exercising.

Underload   The term underload refers to an easier-than-average workout.

Vegans   Vegetarians who eat no animal products whatsoever.

Veins   These vessels carry blood back to the heart. They're a little larger in diameter than arteries. They carry the same amount of blood but at a slower speed.

More resources

Books

Aerobic Fitness
John Mason
(Simon & Schuster, 2001)

Body Blitz
Joanna Hall
(HarperCollins, 2001)

Body for Life
Bill Phillips, Mike D'Orso
(HarperCollins, 2000)

The Complete Book of Running for Women
Claire Kowalchik
(Simon & Schuster, 2000)

The Complete Book of T'ai Chi
Stewart McFarlane
(Dorling Kindersley, 1999)

The Complete Guide to Strength Training
Anita Bean
(A & C Black Limited)

59 Minutes to a Calmer Life
Paul McGee
(Go Mad Books, 2001)

Good Housekeeping Step-by-Step Vegetarian Cook Book
(Ebury Press, 1997)

Jenergy
Jenni Rivett
(HarperCollins, 2001)

KISS Guide to Yoga
Shakta Kaur Khalsa
(Dorling Kindersley, 2001)

KISS Guide to Weight Loss
Barbara Ravage
(Dorling Kindersley, 2001)

Manage Your Mind: The Mental Fitness Guide
Gillian Butler, Tony Hope
(Oxford Paperbacks, 1995)

Matt Roberts 90-day Fitness Plan
Matt Roberts
(Dorling Kindersley, 2001)

The Muscle Fitness Book
Francine St. George
(Simon & Schuster, 2001)

The New York City Ballet Workout
Peter Martins
(William Morrow, 2001)

The Optimum Nutrition Cookbook
Patrick Holford, Judy Ridgway
(Piatkus Books, 2000)

Pilates Gym
Lynne Robinson, Gerry Convey
(Pan, 2001)

The Pilates Body
Brooke Siler
(Michael Joseph, 2000)

Stretching
Bob Anderson
(Shelter Publications, 2000)

Taiji Qigong
Chris Jarmey
(Corpus Publishing, 2001)

3-Minute Abs
Kurt Brungardt
(HarperCollins, 1998)

Yoga and the Quest for the True Self
Stephen Cope
(Bantam Books, 1999)

Magazines

Health & Fitness
Highbury Nexus Limited,
53-79 Highgate Road,
London, NW5 1TW.
Telephone: 020 7331 1000
www.hfonline.co.uk

Men's Fitness
Dennis Publishing,
30 Cleveland Street,
London, W1P 5FF.
Telephone: 020 7907 6000

Muscle & Fitness
Published in the UK by Weider
Publishing Limited,
10 Windsor Court,
Clarence Drive,
Harrogate,
North Yorkshire, HG1 2PE.
Telephone: 01423 504516

UltraFit
Champions House,
5 Princes Street,
Penzance,
Cornwall, TR18 2NL.
Telephone: 01736 350204
www.ultra-fitmagazine.com

Fitness web sites

THERE'S A WEALTH *of information about fitness and health in general on the Web. The following contains some of the most useful and interesting sites. Please note that due to the fast-changing nature of the Net, some of the below may be out of date by the time you read this.*

www.acefitness.org
The official web site of the American Council of Exercise, promoting active, healthy lifestyles and safe fitness products and trends.

www.active.org.uk
Advice on becoming more physically active and building exercise into your daily life from the Health Development Agency's Active for Life site.

www.alexandertechnique.com
Complete guide to the Alexander Technique.

www.amazon.co.uk
Visit this site to buy exercise videos online.

www.benning.army.mil/usapfs/
Doctrine/calisthenics/cal1-6.htm
This page on the US Army's Physical Fitness School has more information on the windmill and links to other exercise pages.

www.bodyactive-superstore.co.uk
Try this online store for equipment, from home cardio machines to chin-up bars to clothing.

www.bodysolid.co.uk
Order fitness equipment, including dumbbells and weight sets online.

www.cardiosport.com
This site of this UK-based heart rate monitor manufacturer offers information about heart-rate monitors and heart rate in general.

www.coolrunning.com/major/97/
training/5k/glen0.htm
Click on this US site for more info on training for a 5k or 10k, or for more running tips.

www.dawp.anet.com
Click here to analyze your diet.

www.fitlinxx.com
Articles on basic fitness, sports training, mind/body and health, and exercise news updates.

www.fitnessdirectory.net/directory/u/
upperleg.html
This page has a diagram of the lower body muscles. Other pages have more diagrams.

www.fitnesslink.com/women/moreabs.shtml
Info on women and abs, plus information on all-around fitness for men and women.

www.fitpro.com/news/exerwat/
exerwat0898.html
All you want to know about biceps and more.

www.ginmiller.com
The official site of US fitness leader Gin Miller.

www.goodgymguide.com.au
A directory of gyms in Australia.

www.gymguide.co.uk
A directory of health, fitness, and sports and leisure clubs in the UK.

www.health.gov.au
Click here for more information about heart health and general health in Australia.

www.healthnet.org.uk
For more information about heart health, check out the site of the Coronary Prevention Group.

www.indiana.edu/~health/weightrn/html
Find out about the benefits of weight training, along with helpful tips for beginners.

www.inliners.co.uk
Find places to go in-line skating in the UK.

www.justmove.org
A health and fitness web site sponsored by the American Heart Association. It has lots of tips and information on health and fitness – specifically cardiovascular health.

www.lotteberk.ch
The web site on Lotte Berk the dancer and the exercise method.

www.massagenetwork.com
Descriptions of the different kinds of massage, and how to find a therapist in your area.

www.netlib.org/misc/jet-lag-diet
This site has a detailed feast, fast, feast diet that is supposed to help you avoid jet lag.

www.ntwrks.com/~mikev/chartla.htm
This web site has a detailed chart of the calorie and fat content of hundreds of foods.

www.philips.co.uk
The Philips company site has info on the Philips Portable Rush Digital Audio Player MP3.

www.primusweb.com/fitnesspartner/ library/activity/garden
Find out how to "circuit train" in your garden.

www.r2bf.co.uk
Buy exercise equipment, including resistance bands, at this site.

www.sweatshop.co.uk
The site for The Sweatshop, a store for running gear. You can order gear or get advice on running, plus useful links.

www.shapeup.org
The Shape Up America site has info about getting in shape and losing weight.

www.ozlines.com.au/heal.htm
An Australian health and fitness directory.

www.sony.com
Click on to the Sony site for more information on the Sony Walkman.

www.speedo.com
The online Speedo swimwear store.

www.sportbreak.co.uk
Click here for information on UK spa and activity holidays.

www.t-mag.com/html/body_123abs.html
Exercises, tips, and training for men. This page is devoted to abdominal workouts.

www.techware.com/health
Give details of your height, weight, age and lifestyle (active, sedentary) and calculate exactly how many calories you need in a day.

www.worldtaichiday.org
The official web site for World Tai Chi and Qigong Day.

www.simplyyoga.co.uk
A source for yoga videos, books, and yoga gear.

Index

Acknowledgments

Author's acknowledgments

The author would like to thank Fit Magazine and FitLinxx.com, especially Lisa Klugman and Rita Trieger. Also, thanks to the Prospect Park YMCA, and all the spas, yoga and Pilates studios and personal trainers who let me explore, ask questions, and stay in shape. Plenty of gratitude to the people at DK who make it all happen, especially Jennifer Williams and LaVonne Carlson-Finnerty. Thanks to editor Eve Steinberg, who asked all the right questions. Finally, thanks to my mother – the sports psychologist and senior tennis champ – Dr. Jo Ann Hundley, Joe Kirstein, Lester and Shelia Parker. And of course, thanks to Ultimate Frisbee champion David Hollander for his advice and moral support.

Publisher's acknowledgments

Dorling Kindersley would like to thank Neal Cobourne for designing the jacket and Melanie Simmonds, David Saldanha, and Hayley Smith for picture research.

Packager's acknowledgments

Cooling Brown would like to thank Pavilion Sports Health & Fitness and Style Fitness Treadmills (www.stylefitness.co.uk). Our thanks also to Barbara Roby and Kate Sheppard for editorial assistance.

Photographers: Steve Gorton, Amanda Heywood, Trevor Morris
Models: Matt Gray, William Heslop, Vicky Kiteley, Lisa Raynbird, Steve Thompson

Index: Patricia Coward

Picture credits
Cooling Brown: 42, 43, 44, 72-73, 74-75, 78, 82, 83, 102-103, 178, 179, 182-183, 184, 186, 187, 188, 194, 195, 197, 198, 199b, 201, 202, 208-209, 210-211, 212t, 213, 214, 215, 220, 221, 222, 225, 226, 227, 229, 230, 231, 265, 266, 267, 268, 270t. **Corbis:** 56, 147 Jim Cummins, 67 M. L. Sinibaldi, 224 Michael Keller, Jose L. Pelaez 263; Mugshots 269; Bettmann 316, 323; Duomo 315. **EyeWire Images:** 14-15, 22, 36, 52, 68, 70, 84, 89, 122, 124, 127, 135, 138, 158, 164, 165, 166t, 167, 168, 170, 172, 192, 204, 232, 233, 234, 236t, 248, 250, 253, 273, 275, 278, 282, 287, 291, 295, 300, 301, 303, 306. **Image 100:** 20, 28, 29, 31, 32, 40t, 55, 57, 58, 64, 77, 96, 317. **Photodisc:** 21, 25, 26, 27, 30, 34, 35, 38, 45, 46, 47, 48, 49, 51, 62, 66, 69, 88, 91, 97, 98, 100, 104, 110, 113, 114, 118, 120, 121, 125, 126, 128, 133, 137, 141, 152, 153, 154, 155, 156, 166, 169, 174, 177, 193, 207, 218, 236, 237, 240, 244, 246, 247, 255, 256, 257, 258, 260, 270, 272, 274, 276, 277, 280, 283, 284, 285, 286, 288, 296, 298, 307, 309, 310, 312, 314, 317, 319 (tl, tc, tr); 320, 324. **Proform:** 93, 95.
Style Fitness: 60, 61, 94.
Illustrations: Dover Publications 24, Peter Cooling 79.
All other images © Dorling Kindersley. For further information see: www.dkimages.com